EVIDENCE-BASED
TREATMENT PLANNING
FOR OBSESSIVE-COMPULSIVE
DISORDER

EVIDENCE-BASED TREATMENT PLANNING FOR OBSESSIVE-COMPULSIVE DISORDER

DVD COMPANION WORKBOOK

ARTHUR E. JONGSMA, JR.
AND
TIMOTHY J. BRUCE

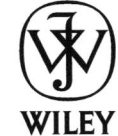

WILEY

John Wiley & Sons, Inc.

Contents

Introduction

This *Workbook* is a companion to the *Evidence-Based Treatment Planning for Obsessive-Compulsive Disorder (OCD)* DVD, which is focused on informing mental health therapists, addiction counselors, and students in these fields about evidence-based psychological treatment planning.

Organization

In this *Workbook* you will find in each chapter:

➤ Summary highlights of content shown in the DVD
➤ Chapter review discussion questions
➤ Chapter review test questions
➤ Chapter references

In appropriate chapters, the references are divided into those for empirical support, those for clinical resources, and those for bibliotherapy resources. Empirical support references are selected studies or reviews of the empirical work that support the efficacy of the empirically supported treatments (ESTs) discussed in the chapter. The clinical resources are books, manuals, or other resources for clinicians that describe the application, or "how-to," of the treatments discussed. The bibliotherapy resources are selected publications and Web sites relevant to the DVD content that may be helpful to clinicians, clients, or laypersons.

Examples of client homework are included at www.wiley.com/go/OCDwb. They are designed to enhance understanding of therapeutic interventions, in addition to being potentially useful clinically.

Appendix A contains an example of an evidence-based treatment plan for OCD. In Appendix B, correct and incorrect answers to all chapter review test questions are explained.

Chapter Points

This DVD is electronically marked with chapter points that delineate the beginning of discussion sections throughout the program. You may skip to any one of these chapter points on the DVD by clicking on the forward arrow. The chapter points for this program are as follows:

➤ Defining OCD
➤ Six Steps in Building a Psychotherapy Treatment Plan
➤ Brief History of the EST Movement
➤ ESTs for OCD
➤ Integrating ESTs for OCD into a Treatment Plan
➤ Common Considerations in Relapse Prevention
➤ An Evidence-Based Treatment Plan for Obsessive-Compulsive Disorder

Series Rationale

Evidence-based practice (EBP) is steadily becoming the standard of mental health care, as it has of medical health care. Borrowing from the Institute of Medicine's definition (Institute of Medicine, 2001), the American Psychological Association (APA) has defined EBP as "the integration of the best available research with clinical expertise in the context of patient characteristics, culture, and preferences" (American Psychological Association Presidential Task Force on Evidence-Based Practice [APA], 2006).

Professional organizations such as the American Psychological Association, the National Association of Social Workers, and the American Psychiatric Association, as well as consumer organizations such the National Alliance for the Mentally Ill (NAMI), are endorsing EBP. At the federal level, a major joint initiative of the National Institute of Mental Health and the Department of Health and Human Services Substance Abuse and Mental Health Services Administration (SAMHSA) focuses on promoting, implementing, and evaluating evidence-based mental health programs and practices within state mental health systems (APA, 2006). In some practice settings, EBP is even becoming mandated. It is clear that the call for evidence-based practice is being increasingly sounded.

Unfortunately, many mental health care providers cannot or do not stay abreast of results from clinical research and how these results can inform their practices. Although it has rightfully been argued that the relevance of some research to the clinician's needs is weak, there are products of clinical research whose efficacy has been well-established and whose effectiveness in the community setting has received support. Clinicians and clinicians-in-training interested in empirically informing their treatments could benefit from educational programs that make this goal more easily attainable.

This series of DVDs and companion workbooks is designed to introduce clinicians and students to the process of empirically informing their psychotherapy treatment plans. The series begins with an introduction to the efforts to identify research-supported treatments and how the products of these efforts can be used to inform treatment planning. The other programs in the series focus on empirically informed treatment planning for each of several commonly seen clinical problems. In each problem-focused DVD, issues involved in defining or diagnosing the presenting problem are reviewed. Research-supported treatments for the problem are described, as well as the process used to identify them. Viewers are then systematically guided through the process of creating a treatment plan, and shown how the plan can be informed by goals, objectives, and interventions consistent with those of the identified research-supported treatments. Example vignettes of selected interventions are also provided.

This series is intended to be educational and informative in nature and not meant to be a substitute for clinical training in the specific interventions discussed and demonstrated. References to empirical support of the treatments described, clinical resource material, and training opportunities are provided.

Presenters

Exhibit I.1   Dr. Tim Bruce and Dr. Art Jongsma

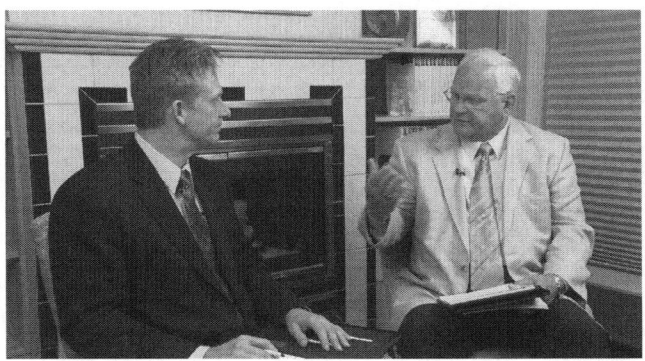

Dr. Art Jongsma is the Series Editor and co-author of the Practice*Planners*® Series published by John Wiley & Sons. He has authored or co-authored more than 40 books in this series. Among the books included in this series are the highly regarded *The Complete Adult Psychotherapy Treatment Planner, The Adolescent Psychotherapy Treatment Planner, The Child Psychotherapy Treatment Planner, and The Addiction Treatment Planner*. All of these books, along with *The Severe and Persistent Mental Illness Treatment Planner, The Family Therapy Treatment Planner, The Couples Psychotherapy Treatment Planner, The Older Adult Psychotherapy Treatment Planner,* and *The Veterans and Active Duty Military Psychotherapy Treatment Planner*, are informed with objectives and interventions that are supported by research evidence.

Dr. Jongsma also created the clinical record management software tool Thera*Scribe*®, which uses point-and-click technology to easily develop, store, and print treatment plans, progress notes, and homework assignments. He has conducted treatment planning and software training workshops for mental health professionals around the world.

Dr. Jongsma's clinical career began as a psychologist in a large private psychiatric hospital. After working in the hospital for about 10 years, he then transitioned to outpatient work in his own private practice clinic, Psychological Consultants, in Grand Rapids, Michigan for 25 years. He has been writing best-selling books and software for mental health professionals since 1995.

Dr. Timothy Bruce is a Professor and Associate Chair of the Department of Psychiatry and Behavioral Medicine at the University of Illinois, College of Medicine in Peoria, Illinois, where he also directs medical student education. He is a licensed clinical psychologist who completed his graduate training at SUNY-Albany, under the mentorship of Dr. David Barlow, and his residency training at Wilford Hall Medical Center, under the direction of Dr. Robert Klepac. In addition to maintaining an active clinical practice at the university, Dr. Bruce has authored numerous publications, including books, professional journal articles, book chapters, and professional educational materials, many on the topic of evidence-based practice. Most recently, he has served as the developmental editor empirically informing Dr. Jongsma's best-selling Practice*Planners*® Series.

Dr. Bruce is also Executive Director of the Center for Evidence-Based Mental Health Practices, a state- and federally funded initiative to disseminate evidence-based psychological and pharmacological practices across Illinois. Highly recognized as an educator, Dr. Bruce has received nearly two dozen awards for his teaching of students and professionals during his career.

References

American Psychological Association Presidential Task Force on Evidence-Based Practice (2006). Evidence-based practice in psychology. *American Psychologist, 61*, 271–285.

Berghuis, D., Jongsma, A., & Bruce, T. (2006). *The severe and persistent mental illness treatment planner* (2nd ed.). Hoboken, NJ: Wiley.

Dattilio, F., Jongsma, A., & Davis, S. (2009). *The family therapy treatment planner* (2nd ed.). Hoboken, NJ: Wiley.

Institute of Medicine. (2001). *Crossing the quality chasm: A new health system for the 21st century.* Washington, DC: National Academy Press

Jongsma, A., Peterson, M., & Bruce, T. (2006). *The complete adult psychotherapy treatment planner* (4th ed.). Hoboken, NJ: Wiley.

Jongsma, A., Peterson, M., McInnis, W., & Bruce, T. (2006a). *The adolescent psychotherapy treatment planner* (4th ed.). Hoboken, NJ: Wiley.

Jongsma, A., Peterson, M., McInnis, W., & Bruce, T. (2006b). *The child psychotherapy treatment planner* (4th ed.). Hoboken, NJ: Wiley.

Moore, B., & Jongsma, A. (2009). *The veterans and active duty military psychotherapy treatment planner.* Hoboken, NJ: Wiley.

Perkinson, R., Jongsma, A., & Bruce, T. (2009). *The addiction treatment planner* (4th ed.). Hoboken, NJ: Wiley.

1

What Is Obsessive–Compulsive Disorder?

Defining Obsessive–Compulsive Disorder

As the name suggests, Obsessive-Compulsive Disorder, or OCD, is defined by the presence of either obsessions or compulsions.

Obsessions

Obsessions are recurrent and persistent thoughts, images, or impulses that are experienced at some time during the disturbance as intrusive and inappropriate, and that cause marked anxiety or distress.

These thoughts, images, or impulses are not simply excessive worries about real-life problems—as seen in Generalized Anxiety Disorder.

Additionally, the OCD sufferer attempts to ignore or suppress the thoughts, impulses, or images, or to neutralize them with some other thought or action.

Lastly, the person recognizes that the obsessional thoughts, impulses, or images are a product of his or her own mind (not imposed from outside, as in thought insertion)—a feature that distinguishes OCD from psychosis.

Obsessions

- Obsessions are recurrent and persistent thoughts, images, or impulses that are intrusive, inappropriate, and cause marked anxiety or distress.
- The obsessions are not simply excessive worries about real-life problems.
- Attempts are made to ignore or suppress such thoughts, impulses, or images or to neutralize them with some other thought or action.
- The person recognizes that the obsessions are a product of his or her own mind (not imposed from the outside, as in thought insertion).

Compulsions

Compulsions are repetitive behaviors or mental acts that the person feels driven to perform in response to an obsession or according to rules that must be applied rigidly. Examples of common behavioral compulsions include repeated handwashing, ordering things, or checking. Examples of common mental compulsions include excessive praying, counting, or repeating words silently.

These behaviors or mental acts are aimed at preventing or reducing distress or preventing some dreaded event or situation; however, they either are not connected in a realistic way with what they are designed to neutralize or prevent, or they are clearly excessive.

Compulsions

- Compulsions are repetitive behaviors or mental acts that the person feels driven to perform in response to an obsession, or according to rules that must be applied rigidly.
- The compulsions are aimed at preventing or reducing distress or preventing some dreaded event or situation; however, they are not connected in a realistic way with what they are designed to neutralize or prevent or are clearly excessive.

Examples of Common Obsessional Themes and Compulsive Actions

OBSESSIONS
- Contamination
- Causing harm
- Need to order things
- Aggressive impulses
- Sexual imagery

COMPULSIONS
- Washing
- Checking
- Arranging things
- Reassurance-seeking
- Hoarding

In OCD, the person has recognized that the obsessions or compulsions are excessive or unreasonable at some point during the course of the disorder, although we'll see later that some individuals with OCD have less insight on this than others. (In addition, this criterion does not apply to children with OCD.)

By definition, all mental disorders cause clinically significant distress or disability. In OCD, the obsessions or compulsions must cause marked distress, be time consuming (take more than one hour per day), or significantly interfere with the person's normal routine, occupational (or academic) functioning, or usual social activities or relationships.

It is important to note that you do not diagnose OCD if an apparent obsession or compulsion is a primary feature of another mental disorder and restricted to it. Examples include the following:

➤ The preoccupation with food within an eating disorder
➤ The compulsive hair pulling within trichotillomania
➤ The concern with appearance within body dysmorphic disorder

And again, as with all mental disorders, you must first rule out that the disturbance is not due to the direct physiological effects of a substance (e.g., a drug of abuse, a medication) or a general medical condition.

Finally in the DSM system, you are asked to specify whether the OCD sufferer has poor insight. This specifier, termed "with poor insight," is used when the person does not recognize, for most of the time during the current episode, that the obsessions and compulsions are excessive or unreasonable.

Diagnostic Criteria for Obsessive–Compulsive Disorder

A. Experiences either obsessions or compulsions

B. At some point during the course of the disorder, the person has recognized that the obsessions or compulsions are excessive or unreasonable (this does not apply to children).

C. The obsessions or compulsions cause marked distress, are time consuming (take more than 1 hour per day), or significantly interfere with the person's normal routine, occupational (or academic) functioning, or usual social activities or relationships.

D. OCD is not diagnosed when an apparent obsession or compulsion is a primary feature of another mental disorder and restricted to it.

E. The disturbance is not due to the direct physiological effects of a substance (e.g., a drug of abuse, a medication) or a general medical condition.

Use the specifier "with poor insight" if the person does not recognize, for most of the time during the current episode, that the obsessions and compulsions are excessive or unreasonable.

From the *Diagnostic and Statistical Manual of Mental Disorders* (APA, 2000).

Chapter Review

1. What are the diagnostic criteria for obsessive-compulsive disorder?

Chapter Review Test Questions

1. Which of the following best reflects the definition of obsessions, according to diagnostic criteria such as those of the DSM?

   A. Recurrent and persistent images
   B. Recurrent and persistent impulses
   C. Recurrent and persistent thoughts
   D. Recurrent and persistent thoughts, images, or impulses

2. Which of the following describes common compulsions?

   A. Aggressive impulses and images
   B. Checking and washing
   C. Contamination fears and washing
   D. Harming fears and reassurance seeking

Chapter Reference

American Psychiatric Association. (2000). *Diagnostic and statistical manual of mental disorders* (4th ed., text revised). Washington, DC: American Psychiatric Association.

2

What Are the Six Steps in Building a Treatment Plan?

Step 1: Identify primary and secondary problems
  ➤ Use evidence-based psychosocial assessment procedures to determine the most significant problem or problems related to current distress, disability, or both.

Step 2: Describe the problem's manifestations (symptom pattern)
  ➤ Note how the problem(s) are evidenced by your particular client. These features may correspond to the diagnostic criteria for the problem.

Step 3: Make a diagnosis based on DSM/ICD criteria
  ➤ Based on an evaluation of the client's complete clinical presentation, determine the appropriate diagnosis using the process and criteria described in the DSM or the ICD.

Step 4: Specify long-term goals
  ➤ These goal statements need not be crafted in measurable terms, but are broader and indicate a desired general positive outcome of treatment.

Step 5: Create short-term objectives
  ➤ Objectives for the client to achieve should be stated in measurable or observable terms so accountability is enhanced.

Step 6: Select therapeutic interventions
  ➤ Interventions are the actions of the clinician within the therapeutic alliance designed to help the client accomplish the treatment objectives. There should be at least one intervention planned for each client objective.

Key Point

One important aspect of effective treatment planning is that each plan should be tailored to the individual client's particular problems and needs. Treatment plans should not be boilerplate, even if clients have similar problems. Consistent with the definition of an evidence-based practice, the individual's strengths and weaknesses, unique stressors, cultural and social network, family circumstances, and symptom patterns must be considered in developing a treatment strategy. Clinicians should rely on their own good clinical judgment and plan a treatment that is appropriate for the distinctive individual with whom they are working.

Chapter Review

1. What are the six steps involved in developing a psychotherapy treatment plan?

Chapter Review Test Questions

1. Persons with obsessive-compulsive disorder may engage in compulsive acts that, although meeting the criteria for a compulsion, are particular to that individual's beliefs regarding how they work. Examples include performing acts in threes, hoarding only certain types of objects, and washing a certain way for a certain length of time. In which step of treatment planning would you record these features of your particular client?

   A. Creating short-term objectives
   B. Describing the problem's manifestations
   C. Identifying the primary problem
   D. Selecting treatment interventions

2. The statement "Discuss with the client how treatment serves as an arena to desensitize learned fear, reality-test obsessional fears and underlying beliefs, and build confidence in managing fears without compulsions," is an example of which of the following features of a treatment plan?

   A. A primary problem
   B. A short-term objective
   C. A symptom manifestation
   D. A treatment intervention

Chapter References

American Psychological Association Presidential Task Force on Evidence-Based Practice. (2006). Evidence-based practice in psychology. *American Psychologist, 61*, 271–185.

Jongsma, A. (2005). Psychotherapy treatment plan writing. In G. P. Koocher, J. C. Norcross, & S. S. Hill (Eds.), *Psychologists' desk reference* (2nd ed., pp. 232–236). New York, NY: Oxford University Press.

Jongsma, A. Peterson, M., & Bruce, T. (2006). *The complete adult psychotherapy treatment planner* (4th ed.). Hoboken, NJ: John Wiley & Sons.

Jongsma, A., Peterson, M., McInnis, W., & Bruce, T. (2006). *The adolescent psychotherapy treatment planner* (4th ed.). Hoboken, NJ: Wiley.

CHAPTER 3

What Is the Brief History of the Empirically Supported Treatments Movement?

In the United States, the effort to identify empirically supported treatments (ESTs) began with an initiative of the American Psychological Association's Division 12— The Society of Clinical Psychology.

In 1993, APA's Division 12 President David Barlow initiated a task group, chaired by Diane Chambless. The group was charged to review the psychotherapy outcome literature to identify psychological treatments whose efficacy had been demonstrated through clinical research. This group was originally called the Task Force on the Promotion and Dissemination of Psychological Procedures, and was later reorganized under the Task Force on Psychological Interventions.

Process Used to Identify Empirically Supported Treatments (ESTs)

Reviewers established two primary sets of criteria for judging the evidence base supporting any particular therapy. One was labeled *well-established*, the other *probably efficacious* (Figure 3.1).

Key Point

Division 12's criteria for a well-established treatment are similar to the standards used by the United States Food and Drug Administration (FDA) to evaluate the safety and efficacy of proposed medications. The FDA requires demonstration that a proposed medication is significantly superior to a nonspecific control treatment (a pill placebo) in at least two randomized controlled trials conducted by independent research groups. Division 12's criteria for a well-established treatment requires the equivalent of this standard as well as other features relevant to judging a psychological treatment's efficacy (e.g., a clear description of the treatment and study participants). By extension, if the FDA were to evaluate psychotherapies using the criteria they use for medication, it would allow sale of those judged to be well-established.

Figure 3.1

Specific Criteria for Well-Established and Probably Efficacious Treatments

Criteria for a Well-Established Treatment

For a psychological treatment to be considered *well-established*, the evidence base supporting it had to be characterized by the following:

I. At least two, good between group design experiments demonstrating efficacy in one or more of the following ways

    A. Superior (statistically significantly so) to pill or psychological placebo or to another treatment

    B. Equivalent to an already established treatment in experiments with adequate sample sizes

OR

II. A large series of single case design experiments ($n > 9$) demonstrating efficacy. These experiments must have:

    A. Used good experimental designs

    B. Compared the intervention to another treatment, as in IA

Further Criteria for Both I and II

III. Experiments must be conducted with treatment manuals.

IV. Characteristics of the client samples must be clearly specified.

V. Effects must have been demonstrated by at least two different investigators or investigating teams.

Criteria for a Probably Efficacious Treatment

For a psychological treatment to be considered *probably efficacious*, the evidence base supporting it had to meet the following criteria:

I. Two experiments showing the treatment is superior (statistically significantly so) to a waiting-list control group.

OR

II. One or more experiments meeting the well-established treatment criteria IA or IB, III, and IV, but not V.

OR

III. A small series of single case design experiments ($n > 3$) otherwise meeting Well-Established Treatment

Adapted from "Update on Empirically Validated Therapies, II," by D. L. Chambless, M. J. Baker, D. H. Baucom, L. E. Beutler, K. S. Calhoun, P. Crits-Christoph, . . . S. R. Woody, 1998, *The Clinical Psychologist, 51*(1), 3–16.

Products of Empirically Supported Treatment Reviews

The products of these reviews can be found in the Division 12 groups' final two reports.

➣ In the first report, 47 ESTs are identified (Chambless et al., 1996).
➣ In the final report, the list had grown to 71 ESTs (Chambless et al., 1998).
➣ In 1999, The Society of Clinical Psychology, Division 12, took full ownership of maintaining the growing list. The current list and information center can be found on its Web site: www.psychologicaltreatment.org.

Around this same time, other groups emerged, using the same or similar criteria, to review literatures related to other populations, problems, and interventions. Examples include the following:

➣ Children (Lonigan & Elbert, 1998)
➣ Pediatric Psychology (Spirito, 1999)
➣ Older Adults (Gatz, 1998)
➣ Adult, Child, Marital, Family Therapy (Kendall & Chambless, 1998)
➣ Psychopharmacology and Psychological Treatments (Nathan & Gorman, 1998; 2002; 2007)

For those interested in comparing and contrasting the criteria used by various review groups, see Chambless and Ollendick (2001).

TherapyAdvisor

Descriptions of the treatments identified through many of these early reviews, as well as references to the empirical work supporting them, clinical resources, and training opportunities, can be found at www.therapyadvisor.com. This resource was developed by Personal Improvement Computer Systems (PICS) with funding from the National Institute of Mental Health and in consultation with members of the original Division 12 task groups. Information found on TherapyAdvisor is provided by the primary author/researcher(s) of the given EST.

Selected Organizational Reviewers of Evidence-Based Psychological Treatments and Practices

➣ The United Kingdom is on the forefront of the effort to identify evidence-based treatments and develop guidelines for practice. The latest products of their work can be found at the Web site for the National Institute for Health and Clinical Excellence (NICE): www.nice.org.uk.

➢ The Substance Abuse and Mental Health Service Administration, or SAMHSA, has an initiative to evaluate, identify, and provide information on various mental health practices. Their work, entitled "The National Registry of Evidence-based Programs and Practices or NREPP," can be found online at www.nrepp .samhsa.gov.

➢ The Agency for Health Care Policy and Research, now called the Agency for Healthcare Research and Quality (AHRQ), has established guidelines and criteria for identifying evidence-based practices and provides links to evidence-based clinical practice guidelines for various medical and mental health problems at www.ahrq.gov/clinic/epcix.htm.

Chapter Review

1. How did Division 12 of the APA identify ESTs?
2. What are the primary differences between well-established and probably efficacious criteria used to identify ESTs?
3. Where can information about ESTs and evidence-based practices be found?

Chapter Review Test Questions

1. Which statement best describes the process used to identify ESTs?

   A. Consumers of mental health services nominated therapies
   B. Experts came to a consensus based on their experiences with the treatments
   C. Researchers submitted their works
   D. Task groups reviewed the literature using clearly defined selection criteria for ESTs

2. Based on the differences in their criteria, in which of the following ways are well-established treatments different than those classified as probably efficacious?

   A. Only the probably efficacious criteria allowed the use of single case design experiments.
   B. Only the well-established criteria allowed studies comparing the treatment to a psychological placebo.
   C. Only the well-established criteria required demonstration by at least two different, independent investigators or investigating teams.
   D. Only the well-established criteria allowed studies comparing the treatment to a pill placebo.

Chapter References

Chambless, D. L., & Ollendick, T. H. (2001). Empirically supported psychological interventions: Controversies and evidence. *Annual Review of Psychology, 52,* 685–716.

Chambless, D. L., Sanderson, W. C., Shoham, V., Bennett Johnson, S., Pope, K. S., Crits-Christoph, P., . . . McCurry, S. (1996). An update on empirically validated therapies. *The Clinical Psychologist, 49,* 5–18.

Chambless, D. L., Baker, M. J., Baucom, D. H., Beutler, L. E., Calhoun, K. S., Crits-Christoph, P., . . . Woody, S. R. (1998). Update on empirically validated therapies, II. *The Clinical Psychologist, 51,* 3–16.

Gatz, M., Fiske, A., Fox, L. S., Kaskie, B., Kasl-Godley, J. E., McCallum, T., & Wetherell, J. (1998). Empirically validated psychological treatments for older adults. *Journal of Mental Health and Aging, 41,* 9–46.

Kendall, P. C., & Chambless, D. L. (Eds.). (1998). Empirically supported psychological therapies [special issue]. *Journal of Consulting and Clinical Psychology, 66 (3),* 151–162.

Lonigan, C. J., & Elbert, J. C. (Eds.). (1998). Empirically supported psychosocial interventions for children [special issue]. *Journal of Clinical Child Psychology, 27,* 138–226.

Nathan, P. E., & Gorman, J. M. (Eds.). (1998). *A guide to treatments that work.* New York, NY: Oxford University Press.

Nathan, P. E., & Gorman, J. M. (Eds.). (2002). *A guide to treatments that work* (2nd ed.). New York, NY: Oxford University Press.

Nathan, P. E., & Gorman, J. M. (Eds.). (2007). *A guide to treatments that work* (3rd ed.). New York, NY: Oxford University Press.

Spirito, A. (Ed.). (1999). Empirically supported treatments in pediatric psychology [special issue]. *Journal of Pediatric Psychology, 24,* 87–174.

4

What Are the Identified Empirically Supported Treatments for Obsessive–Compulsive Disorder?

Empirically informing a treatment plan as described in this series involves integrating those aspects of empirically supported treatments (ESTs) into each step of the treatment planning process discussed previously. There are several independent reviews of the psychotherapy outcome literature for the treatment of OCD that have identified either empirically supported treatments or evidence-based practice guidelines. These include APA's Division 12, Franklin and Foa in Nathan & Gorman's series *A Guide to Treatments that Work*, NICE in the United Kingdom, and others. There is also great uniformity in the conclusions drawn from these reviews regarding which treatments have demonstrated efficacy for OCD.

The Society of Clinical Psychology

Using their selection process discussed previously, APA's Division 12 (The Society of Clinical Psychology) has identified exposure and response (or ritual) prevention (ERP) and cognitive therapy (CT) as two therapeutic approaches that have met their criteria for a well-established EST.

Well-Established ESTs for OCD

- Exposure and Response (or Ritual) Prevention
- Cognitive Therapy

See www.psychologicaltreatments.org.

Exposure and Response (or Ritual) Prevention (ERP)

As with its application to other anxiety disorders, exposure asks clients to engage repeatedly in what they fear, allowing the learned fear to extinguish over time.

With OCD, it has been found that exposure works best when used with response (or ritual) prevention. Generally speaking, response prevention asks the client to refrain from engaging in their rituals once they have begun exposure to the triggers that have previously prompted them.

Exposures are typically guided by a hierarchy in which less feared activities are conducted first. Imaginal exposure, live (or *in vivo*) exposure, or both may be used in treating OCD. Imaginal exposure typically involves imagining an obsessive thought or image or the feared consequences of them, allowing the emotion attached to the image to weaken. For example, a client who obsesses that loved ones may die if the client should neglect to check potential household hazards repeatedly might be asked to vividly imagine the deaths, while refraining from the mental ritual. The purpose of this type of exposure is to reduce the fear of the thought or image.

Exposure *in vivo* involves asking the client to actually engage in the activity they fear. For example, a client who fears contamination in a bathroom might be asked to touch something they feel is contaminated while refraining from ritualized handwashing. The therapist would encourage the client to continue the exposure during the session until anxiety associated with it waned. They would then repeat this exercise until there was evidence of extinction from session to session.

Exposure and Response (or Ritual) Prevention (ERP)

- Exposure asks clients to engage repeatedly in what they fear, allowing the learned fear to extinguish over time.
- Response prevention asks the client to refrain from engaging in their compulsive rituals.
- Exposures are typically guided by a fear hierarchy.
- Imaginal exposure, live (or *in vivo*) exposure, or both may be used in treating OCD.
- Imaginal exposure typically involves imagining an obsessive thought or image or the feared consequences of them.
- Exposure *in vivo* involves asking the client to engage in the actual activity they fear.

Cognitive Therapy for OCD

Cognitive therapy (CT) for OCD derives from a model in which biased cognitive appraisals of oneself, the environment, and/or the future, lead the person to emotional reactions and behavioral actions that can be distressing and maladaptive.

Identifying and changing those appraisals to facilitate better adaptation is the target of the therapy.

Cognitive biases commonly addressed in OCD include the following: overestimating the likelihood of catastrophic outcomes to everyday events; interpreting the presence of obsessions as indicating some personal flaw or troubling intention (e.g., the "thinking is the same as doing" bias, also known as the "thought-action fusion"); and holding an inflated sense of personal responsibility over events that may cause harm to oneself or others.

Cognitive therapy helps clients learn the connections among one's thoughts, emotions, and actions. It begins by teaching the client the connection between thinking and feeling. Clients learn how to identify biased thinking, challenge its validity, develop alternative appraisals, and validate either the fearful or alternative appraisals by converting them into predictions and testing them in reality through exercises called behavioral experiments.

Dialogue with the therapist, as well as in-session and between-session exercises, are the primary vehicles used in CT.

Cognitive therapy techniques, along with exposure and response prevention, are often integrated in a single therapy commonly referred to as cognitive behavioral therapy (CBT) involving ERP.

Cognitive Theory and Therapy

- *Cognitive Theory*: Biased cognitive appraisals lead to emotional reactions and behavioral actions that may be distressing and maladaptive.
- *Cognitive Therapy*: Identifies and changes cognitive appraisals to facilitate better adaptation.

Common Cognitive Biases in OCD

- Overestimating the likelihood of catastrophic outcomes
- Interpreting the presence of obsessions as indicating some personal flaw or troubling intention (thought-action fusion, or "thinking is the same as doing")
- Holding an inflated sense of personal responsibility over events that may cause harm to oneself or others

> ## Cognitive Therapy Process
>
> - Learn the connection between one's thoughts, emotions, and actions
> - Identify biases in thinking
> - Challenge the validity of appraisals
> - Develop alternative, unbiased appraisals
> - Test cognitive appraisals through behavioral experiments
> - Identify and challenge underlying assumptions

Other Reviewers of the OCD Treatment Outcome Literature

In their review of the OCD treatment outcome literature, published in the most recent edition of Nathan and Gorman's *A Guide to Treatments That Work*, Franklin and Foa (2007) identified CBT involving ERP as a well-established treatment for OCD, citing many randomized controlled trials supporting its efficacy. These authors noted that although CT for OCD has a smaller and more recent evidence base than CBT with ERP, it too can be considered a well-established treatment option.

Evidence-based practice guidelines published by organizational reviewers such as NICE in the United Kingdom (see www.nice.org.uk) and the AHRQ in the United States (see www.ahrq.gov/clinic/epcix.htm) also recommend CBT including ERP as the first-line intervention for OCD. These guidelines suggest that cognitive therapy should be considered when clients will not participate in exposure.

> ## Modalities of Delivery
>
> - CBT for OCD is usually conducted on an outpatient basis twice a week. The total number of sessions differs depending on severity, but averages 12 to 16.
> - CBT for OCD has also been used successfully as an intensive inpatient treatment, typically involving sessions five days a week for three or more weeks.
> - CBT for OCD has also been conducted successfully in a group format, a modality commonly used for less severe versions of the disorder.

Conclusion

For our purposes in demonstrating evidence-based treatment planning, we use the definition of an evidence-based practice advanced by the American Psychological

Association, which states that it is "the integration of the best available research with clinical expertise, in the context of patient characteristics, culture, and preferences."

Conclusions from reviewers of the treatment outcome literature for OCD as well as recommendations from developers of evidence-based practice guidelines suggest that CBT including ERP is a well-established treatment for OCD and an appropriate first-line consideration in an evidence-based approach to treating OCD psychotherapeutically.

Chapter Review

1. As presented in this chapter, what are the empirically supported psychological treatments for OCD?

Chapter Review Test Questions

1. Cognitive behavioral therapy (CBT) that includes which of the following is a well-established treatment for OCD and the recommended first-line psycho-therapeutic treatment option in evidence-based practice guidelines?

   A. Exposure and response prevention (ERP)
   B. Psychoeducation (PE)
   C. Relaxation training (RT)
   D. Systematic desensitization (SD)

2. Asking a client with OCD to stop or limit compulsive rituals associated with an exposure is known as which of the following?

   A. Behavioral experiment
   B. Cognitive restructuring
   C. Limit setting
   D. Response prevention

Selected Chapter References

Empirical Support

Abramowitz, J. S. (1996). Variants of exposure and response prevention in the treatment of obsessive-compulsive disorder: A meta-analysis. *Behavior Therapy, 27,* 583–600.

Abramowitz, J. S. (1997). Effectiveness of psychological and pharmacological treatments for obsessive-compulsive disorder: A quantitative review. *Journal of Consulting and Clinical Psychology, 65,* 44–52.

Abramowitz, J. S., Foa, E. B., & Franklin, M. E. (2003). Exposure and ritual prevention for obsessive-compulsive disorder: Effects of intensive versus twice-weekly sessions. *Journal of Consulting and Clinical Psychology, 71*, 394–398.

Emmelkamp, P. M. G., & Beens. H. (1991). Cognitive therapy with obsessive-compulsive disorder: A comparative evaluation. *Behaviour Research and Therapy, 18*, 61–66.

Emmelkamp, P. M. G., Visser, S., & Hoekstra, R. J. (1988). Cognitive therapy vs. exposure *in vivo* in the treatment of obsessive-compulsives. *Cognitive Therapy and Research, 12*, 103–114.

Fals-Stewart, W., Marks, A. P., & Schafer, J. (1993). A comparison of behavioral group therapy and individual behavior therapy in treating obsessive-compulsive disorder. *Journal of Nervous and Mental Disease, 181*, 189–193.

Foa, E. B., Liebowitz, M. R., Kozak, M. J., Davies, S. O., Campeas, R., Franklin, M. E., . . . Tu, X. (2005). Randomized placebo-controlled trial of exposure and ritual prevention, clomipramine, and their combination in the treatment of obsessive compulsive disorder. *American Journal of Psychiatry, 162*, 151–161.

Foa, E. B., Steketee, G., Grayson, J. B., Turner, R. M., & Latimer, P. (1984). Deliberate exposure and blocking of obsessive-compulsive rituals: Immediate and long-term effects. *Behavior Therapy, 15*, 450–472.

Foa, E. B., Steketee, G. S., & Milby, J. B. (1980). Differential effects of exposure and response prevention in obsessive-compulsive washers. *Journal of Consulting and Clinical Psychology, 48*, 71–79.

Foa, E. B., Steketee, G., Turner, R. M., & Fischer, S. C. (1980). Effects of imaginal exposure to feared disasters in obsessive-compulsive checkers. *Behaviour Research and Therapy, 18*, 449–455.

Franklin, M. E., Abramowitz, J. S., Kozak, M. J., Levitt, J. T., & Foa, E. B. (2000). Effectiveness of exposure and ritual prevention for obsessive-compulsive disorder: Randomized compared with nonrandomized samples. *Journal of Consulting and Clinical Psychology, 68*, 594–602.

Franklin, M. E., & Foa, E. B. (2007). Cognitive behavioral treatment of obsessive-compulsive disorder. In P. E. Nathan & J. M. Gorman (Eds.), *A guide to treatments that work* (3rd ed., pp. 431–446). New York, NY: Oxford University Press.

Freeston, M. H., Ladouceur, R., Gagnon, F., Thibodeau, N., Rheaume, J., Letarte, H., & Bujold, A. (1997). Cognitive-behavioral treatment of obsessive thoughts: A controlled study. *Journal of Consulting and Clinical Psychology, 65*, 405–413.

Lindsay, M., Crino, R., & Andrews, G. (1997). Controlled trial of exposure and response prevention in obsessive-compulsive disorder. *British Journal of Psychiatry, 171*, 135–139.

Marks, I. M., Lelliott, P., Basoglu, M., Noshirvani, H., Monteiro, W., Cohen, D., & Kasvikis, Y. (1988). Clomipramine, self exposure and therapist-aided exposure for obsessive compulsive rituals. *British Journal of Psychiatry, 152,* 522–534.

Van Blakom, A. J. L. M., van Oppen, P., Vermeulen, A. W. A., & van Dyck, R. (1994). A meta-analysis on the treatment of obsessive compulsive disorder: A comparison of antidepressants, behavior, and cognitive therapy. *Clinical Psychology Review, 14,* 359–381.

Van Oppen, P., de Haan, E., Van Balkom, A. J. L. M., & Spinhoven, P. (1995). Cognitive therapy and exposure *in vivo* in the treatment of obsessive-compulsive disorder. *Behaviour Research and Therapy, 33,* 379–390.

Whittal, M. L., Thordarson, D. S., & McLean, P. D. (2005). Treatment of obsessive-compulsive disorder: Cognitive behavior therapy vs. exposure and response prevention. *Behaviour Research and Therapy. 43,* 1559–1576.

Whittal, M. L., Robichaud, M., Thordarson, D. S., & McLean, P. D. (2008). Group and individual treatment of obsessive-compulsive disorder using cognitive therapy and exposure plus response prevention: A 2-year follow-up of two randomized trials. *Journal of Consulting and Clinical Psychology, 76,* 1003–1014.

Clinical Resources

Beck, A. T., Emery, G., & Greenberg, R. L. (1990). *Anxiety disorders and phobias: A cognitive perspective.* New York, NY: Basic Books.

Brown, T. A., DiNardo, P. A., & Barlow, D. H. (2006). *Anxiety disorders interview schedule, adult version (ADIS-IV): Client interview schedule.* New York, NY: Oxford University Press.

Clark, D. A. (2006). *Cognitive-behavioral therapy for OCD.* New York, NY: Guilford Press.

Goodman, W. K., Price, L. H., Rasmussen, S. A., Mazure, C., Delgado, P., Heninger, G. R., & Charney, D. S. (1989a). The Yale-Brown Obsessive-Compulsive Scale II. Validity. *Archives of General Psychiatry, 46,* 1012–1016.

Goodman, W. K., Price, L. H., Rasmussen, S. A., Mazure, C., Fleishmann, R. L., Hill, C. L., . . . Charney, D. S. (1989b). The Yale-Brown Obsessive-Compulsive Scale I. Development, use, and reliability. *Archives of General Psychiatry, 46,* 1006–1011.

Kozak, M., & Foa, E. (2005). *Mastery of obsessive-compulsive disorder: A cognitive behavioral approach* (therapist guide). New York, NY: Oxford University Press.

McGinn, L., & Sanderson, W. C. (1999). *Treatment of obsessive-compulsive disorder.* Northvale, NJ: Jason Aronson, Inc.

Salkovskis, P. M., & Kirk, J. (1997). Obsessive-compulsive disorder. In D. M. Clark & C. G. Fairburn (Eds.), *Science and practice of cognitive behaviour therapy* (pp. 129–168). Oxford, England: Oxford University Press.

Steketee, G. (1999). *Overcoming obsessive-compulsive disorder A behavioral and cognitive protocol for the treatment of OCD* (therapist protocol). Oakland, CA: New Harbinger.

Steketee, G., & Frost, R. O. (2006). *Compulsive hoarding and acquiring* (therapist guide). New York, NY: Oxford University Press.

Waite, P., & Williams, T. (2009). *Obsessive compulsive disorder: Cognitive behaviour therapy with children and young people.* New York, NY: Routledge.

Bibliotherapy Resources

Abramowitz, J. S. (2009). *Getting over OCD: A 10-step workbook for taking back your life.* New York, NY: Guilford Press.

Carmin, C. N. (2009). *Obsessive-compulsive disorder demystified: An essential guide for understanding and living with OCD.* Philadelphia, PA: De Capo Press.

Foa, E., & Kozak, M. (2004). *Mastery of obsessive-compulsive disorder* (client workbook). New York, NY: Oxford University Press.

Foa, E. B., & Wilson, R. (2001). *Stop obsessing!* (revised ed.). New York, NY: Bantam Books.

Hyman, B. M., & Pedrick, C. (2005). *The OCD workbook* (2nd. ed.). Oakland, CA: New Harbinger Publications.

Landsman, K. J., Rupertus, K. M., and Pedrick, C. (2005). *Loving someone with OCD: Help for you and your family.* Oakland, CA: New Harbinger Publications.

Munford, P. (2004). *Overcoming compulsive checking: Free your mind from OCD.* Oakland, CA: New Harbinger Publications.

Munford, P. (2005). *Overcoming compulsive washing: Free your mind from OCD.* Oakland, CA: New Harbinger Publications.

Neziroglu, F., Bubrick, J., & Yaryura-Tobias, J. A. (2004). *Overcoming compulsive hoarding: Why you save & how you can stop.* Oakland, CA: New Harbinger Publications.

Purdon, C., & Clark, D. A. (2005). *Overcoming obsessive thoughts: How to gain control of your OCD.* Oakland, CA: New Harbinger Publications.

Steketee, G. (1999). *Overcoming obsessive-compulsive disorder: A behavioral and cognitive protocol for the treatment of OCD* (client manual). Oakland, CA: New Harbinger.

Steketee, G., & Frost, R. O. (2006). *Compulsive hoarding and acquiring* (client workbook). New York, NY: Oxford University Press.

Workshop and Training Opportunities

➤ The Center for Treatment and Study of Anxiety, University of Pennsylvania, Philadelphia, PA; see the Web site at www.med.upenn.edu/ctsa/workshops_ocd.html.

➤ The American Institute of Cognitive Therapy, New York, NY; see the Web site at www.cognitivetherapynyc.com.

➤ The Beck Institute; see the Web site at www.beckinstitute.org.

➤ The annual meeting of the Association for Behavioral and Cognitive Therapies; see the Web site at www.abct.org.

CHAPTER 5

How Do You Integrate Empirically Supported Treatments Into Treatment Planning?

Construction of an empirically informed treatment plan for obsessive-compulsive disorder (OCD) involves integrating objectives and treatment interventions consistent with identified empirically supported treatments (ESTs) into a client's treatment plan after you have determined that the client's primary problem fits those described in the target population of the EST research. Of course, implementing ESTs must be done in consideration of important client, therapist, and therapeutic relationship factors—consistent with APA's definition of evidence-based practice.

Definitions

The behavioral definition statements describe *how the problem manifests itself in the client*. Although there are several common features of OCD, the behavioral definition of OCD for your client will be unique and specific to him or her. Your assessment will need to identify which features best characterize your client's presentation. Accordingly, the *behavioral definition* of your treatment plan is tailored to your individual client's clinical picture. When the primary problem reflects a recognized psychiatric diagnosis, the behavioral definition statements are usually closely aligned with diagnostic criteria such as those provided in the DSM or ICD. Examples of common OCD definition statements are the following:

➤ Intrusive, recurrent, and unwanted thoughts, images, or impulses that distress and/or interfere with the client's daily routine, job performance, or social relationships
➤ Failed attempts to ignore or control these thoughts or impulses or neutralize them with other thoughts and actions
➤ Recognition that obsessive thoughts are a product of his/her own mind

> ➤ Repetitive and/or excessive mental or behavioral actions done to neutralize or prevent discomfort or some dreaded outcome
> ➤ Recognition of repetitive thoughts and/or behaviors as being excessive and unreasonable, not realistic worries about life's problems
> ➤ Others

Note the focus on intrusive thoughts or impulsive behaviors and then the failed attempts to control them. Additionally, to settle on the OCD diagnosis, you should find that the client understands that the intrusive thoughts come from within and not from some outside source, as with psychosis. The performance of repetitive actions to prevent some dreaded outcome is common. And the client must realize that his or her repetitive behaviors are unreasonable.

Goals

Goals are broad statements describing what you and the client would like the result of therapy to be. One statement may suffice, but more than one can be used in the treatment plan. Examples of common goal statements for OCD are the following:

> ➤ Reduce the frequency, intensity, and duration of obsessions and compulsive behaviors
> ➤ Reduce time involved with or interference from obsessions and compulsions
> ➤ Function daily at a consistent level with minimal interference from obsessions and compulsions
> ➤ Others

Objectives and Interventions

Objectives are statements that describe *small, observable steps the client must achieve* toward attaining the goal of successful treatment. Intervention statements describe the *actions taken by the therapist* to assist the client in achieving his/her objectives. Each objective must be paired with at least one intervention.

Assessment

All approaches to quality treatment start with a thorough assessment of the nature and history of the client's presenting problems. EST approaches to treatment rely on a thorough psychosocial assessment of the nature, history, and severity of the problem as experienced by the client.

Table 5.1 contains examples of assessment objectives and interventions for OCD.

Table 5.1   Assessment Objectives and Interventions

Objectives	Interventions
1. Describe the history and nature of OCD symptoms.	1. Focus on developing a level of trust with the client; provide support and empathy to encourage the client to feel safe in expressing his/her OCD symptoms. 2. Assess the client's frequency, intensity, duration, and history of obsessions and compulsions (e.g., *The Anxiety Disorders Interview Schedule for the DSM-IV* by DiNardo, Brown, & Barlow).
2. Complete psychological tests designed to assess and track the nature and severity of obsessions and compulsions.	1. Administer an objective test of OCD symptoms to further assess its depth and breadth (e.g., *The Yale-Brown Obsessive Compulsive Scale* by Goodman et al.)
3. Obtain a complete physical evaluation to rule out medica - and substance-related etiologies for anxiety symptoms.	1. Refer the client to a general physician for a complete physical examination to evaluate for any organic basis for the anxiety. 2. Assist the client in following up on the recommendations from a physical evaluation, including medications, lab work, or specialty assessments.
4. Cooperate with a medication evaluation.	1. Arrange for an evaluation as to the need for psychotropic medication to reduce anxiety and control OCD symptoms.

Psychoeducation

A typical feature of many ESTs for OCD is initial and ongoing psychoeducation. A common emphasis is helping the client learn about OCD, the treatment, and its rationale. Often, books or other reading material are recommended to the client to supplement psychoeducation done in session. It is important to instill hope in the client and have him or her on board as a partner in the treatment process. With ESTs, discussing their demonstrated efficacy with the client can facilitate this.

Table 5.2 contains examples of a psychoeducational objective and interventions for OCD.

Table 5.2   Psychoeducational Objective and Interventions

Objective	Interventions
5. Verbalize an understanding of the rationale for treatment of OCD.	1. Assign the client to read psychoeducational chapters of books or treatment manuals on the rationale for exposure and ritual prevention therapy and/or cognitive restructuring for OCD (e.g., *Mastery of Obsessive-Compulsive Disorder* by Kozak & Foa; or *Stop Obsessing* by Foa & Wilson or *Brain Lock: Free Yourself from Obsessive-Compulsive Behavior* by Schwartz). 2. Discuss how treatment serves as an arena to desensitize learned fear, reality-test obsessional fears and underlying beliefs, and build confidence in managing fears without compulsions (see *Mastery of Obsessive-Compulsive Disorder* by Kozak & Foa).

Assessment/Psychoeducation Review

1. What are common emphases of initial psychoeducation?

Assessment/Psychoeducation Review Test Question

1. At what point in therapy is psychoeducation typically conducted?

    A. At the end of therapy
    B. During the assessment phase
    C. During the initial treatment session
    D. Throughout therapy

Cognitive Therapy for OCD

Cognitive therapy (CT) derives from a model in which biased cognitive appraisals of oneself, the environment, and/or the future lead the person to emotional reactions and behavioral actions that can be distressing and maladaptive. Cognitive therapy helps clients learn the connection between one's thoughts, emotions, and actions. Identifying and changing those appraisals to facilitate better adaptation is the target of the therapy.

CT begins by helping the client to identify biased thinking, challenge its validity, develop alternative appraisals, and test the appraisals or predictions in reality through exercises called behavioral experiments. Dialogues with the therapist, as well as in-session and between-session homework exercises, are the primary techniques used in cognitive therapy. Cognitive biases commonly addressed in OCD include overestimating the likelihood of catastrophic outcomes to everyday events (e.g., not washing will result in contamination), interpreting the presence of obsessions as indicating some personal flaw or troubling intention (e.g., if I think of harming someone I must want to do it and may), and holding an inflated sense of personal responsibility over events that may cause harm to oneself or others (e.g., I have to ritualize or the feared outcome will happen).

Key Points

ELEMENTS OF THE COGNITIVE THERAPY PROCESS

- Learn the connection between one's thoughts, emotions, and actions
- Identify biases in thinking
- Challenge validity of appraisals
- Develop alternative appraisals
- Test new thoughts through behavioral experiments
- Examine underlying assumptions of fearful beliefs

Key Points

COMMON COGNITIVE BIASES IN OCD

- Overestimating the likelihood and severity of feared outcomes
- Interpreting the presence of obsessions as indicating some personal flaw or troubling intention
- Holding an inflated sense of personal responsibility over events that may cause harm to oneself or others

---

Table 5.3 contains examples of a cognitive therapy objective and interventions for OCD.

Table 5.3   Cognitive Therapy Objective and Interventions

Objective	Interventions
7. Identify and replace biased, fearful self-talk and beliefs.	1. Explore the client's biased schema and self-talk that mediate his/her obsessional fears and compulsive behavior; assist him/her in generating thoughts that correct for the biases; use behavioral experiments to test fearful versus alternative predictions (see *Mastery of Obsessive-Compulsive Disorder* by Kozak & Foa; or *Obsessive-Compulsive Disorder* by Salkovskis & Kirk).
	2. Assign the client a homework exercise in which he/she identifies fearful self-talk, tests (through behavioral experiments) the predictions from these dysfunctional thoughts, and creates reality-based alternatives; review and reinforce success, providing corrective feedback toward improvement.

Demonstration Vignette
Cognitive Therapy

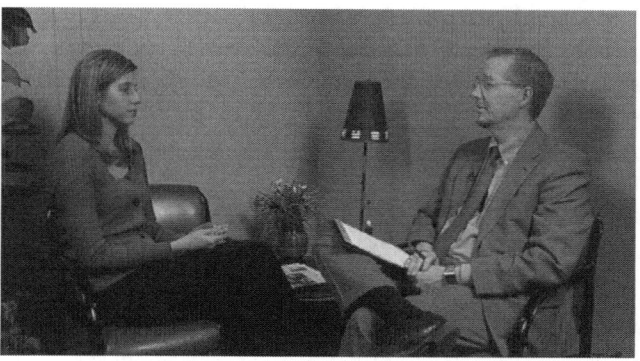

(continued)

Here we present the transcript of the dialogue depicted in the cognitive therapy vignette.

Therapist: You've done a good job with the diary of your thoughts, Jan. So the chance that you might have to use a restroom other than the one you have at home brings on this fearful self-talk.

Client: Yeah. I try to just use my own, but sometimes I have to use a public restroom, and that's hard for me.

Therapist: Most of the self-talk examples are about how you need to avoid getting germs on you. And if you do, your concern is . . . ?

Client: Getting sick.

Therapist: Of course. What does getting sick mean to you?

Client: I don't know. I don't like to think about it. It's awful. I hate the thought of it.

Therapist: I understand. It is important that we talk about it some here though.

Client: I know.

Therapist: Most people don't like getting sick. For awhile you feel bad. It takes you out of your day-to-day life. For you, it's more than that?

Client: I guess. I just don't like it. I guess I'm afraid of the consequences of getting sick?

Therapist: Something worse?

Client: It sounds silly, but yeah . . . like . . . like dying or something.

Therapist: Okay. That's not silly but it may be unrealistic. It's a fear . . . people have fears. Sometimes our fears are realistic, and the anxiety we feel helps keep us from danger. Other times our fears are unfounded, so therefore the anxiety is not helpful. Your mind is thinking that germs will lead to you becoming ill, so you avoid germs at all cost, but what if that belief is not accurate?

Client: How do you know the difference, whether the fear is realistic or not?

Therapist: Good question. First, we need to know exactly what the fear is saying. Then we need to see if what it is saying makes sense in reality. Let's explore further what it's saying to you, so to speak.

Therapist: So we now have a good picture of what this fear is saying to you, when you're anxious. It's saying, "I can't get the germs on me. They'll get inside me and make me sick. If I were sick, it would be horrible. I might even die."

Client: When I hear it like that it sounds kinda crazy.

Therapist: Well, it's important to hear it the way it sounds. Sometimes it gives us perspective. When you heard it this way, you said it sounds crazy. What about it strikes you as crazy?

Client: I don't know. I mean I can see I'm probably not going to die, but I can't help it. It's like it has control over me.

Therapist: I understand. So when you say "crazy" you mean that the fearful self-talk is exaggerating the likelihood of death. You can see this logically, but it's hard to fully believe it, right?

Client: Yeah. I can see logically that I probably won't die. It's just hard to convince myself of that when I'm scared.

Therapist: That's true. Strong emotions, like when you feel really scared, can be very convincing. When we feel a strong emotion like fear, or depression, or anger for that matter, it sometimes makes what we are thinking at the moment seem truer. For example, when people are really angry, have you found that they aren't really open to alternative points of view at that moment?

Client: Yeah, to say the least.

Therapist: Right, you've seen this. What they are thinking at the moment is very convincing to them, but does that make it true? Ever known someone to be angry, but they don't know the whole story? I mean their anger is based on just part of the story or even misinformation?

Client: Yeah. I suppose that's the case most of the time when you're angry.

Therapist: Perhaps. Do you see that feeling something strongly can make what we're thinking at the moment very convincing . . . but the feeling doesn't necessarily mean it's true, does it?

Client: No, I guess not. I guess if you don't know the whole story.

Therapist: So let's look at what your fear is telling you and see if it's telling you the whole story.

Client: All right.

Therapist: So, let's imagine that every time this fearful voice decides to tell you these things, it has to make a prediction of what will actually happen. So what would the fear predict in this case: "If I use a public restroom, I'm going to . . . ?

Client: Um . . . get sick?

Therapist: Sure, that's what it is saying. And getting sick would lead to what?

Client: Well, I guess dying.

Therapist: It says that sometimes, doesn't it? Also feeling awful?

Client: Yeah.

Therapist: You see we're forcing it to make predictions, and this is what it predicts. Every time you've felt anxious about being contaminated, the fearful voice is essentially making a prediction that you are likely to get sick . . . that it will be awful . . . and that you could die. Do you agree that this is the prediction?

Client: Yeah, if you are forced to make a prediction, okay. It sounds a little dramatic when you think of it that way.

Therapist: Right, you're getting that perspective thing again.

Client: [smiles]

Therapist: But, this is what it's saying, correct?

Client: Yeah.

Therapist: Now, let's look at whether it's telling the truth. If it is, it should be predicting pretty accurately.

Client: All right.

Therapist: How many times do you think the thought that you might be contaminated has crossed your mind?

Client: Oh wow, I don't know . . . probably thousands . . . millions.

Therapist: So, if the prediction is right, then how many times should you have gotten sick? And how many times did you actually get sick? Shouldn't they be the same?

(continued)

Client:	I see. No, of course I've not been sick a thousand times, maybe just a few times in the last three or four years.
Therapist:	Good. You're getting it. By challenging the voice, when you make it predict, you've learned, in reality, that the fear predicts sickness way more than it actually occurs.
Client:	Yeah, it does.
Therapist:	That's the overestimation bias we've talked about. But it has been right about getting sick a few times, hasn't it?
Client:	Yeah, I've been sick before.
Therapist:	Right, but all the bad consequences of getting sick?
Client:	Right, I'm still here.
Therapist:	Our self-talk influences what we feel and how strong we feel it. Your self-talk has been overestimating the likelihood of getting sick . . . and it clearly overestimated how severe your sickness would be. It hasn't resulted in your death or need for hospitalization. Looking at the evidence from your life, how would you finish this sentence: "Getting sick isn't pleasant, but it's not . . . ?"
Client:	Going to kill me.
Therapist:	Exactly. So the realistic self-talk messages you can give yourself to replace the exaggerated ones are: I'm probably not going to get sick from these germs. And if I do get sick it's not going to kill me. That's a prediction that has been proven in the past. I think for you to believe it again, we're going to have to test it. Let's talk about that.

Critique of the Cognitive Therapy Demonstration Vignette

The following points were made in the critique:

a. Notice how the therapist led the client to break down her self-talk associated with her fear and even to begin to challenge it.

b. The therapist did a nice job of pointing out how strong feelings convince us that our perspective is true and accurate when it often is distorted by the strong feeling such as anger or fear.

c. The connection between thoughts and emotions (fears) was taught.

d. Believing positive, alternative ways of thinking about stressful situations rarely comes from just talking about the alternatives; behavioral experiments are needed to have the client test the validity of the alternatives in daily living.

e. Prescribing a behavioral experiment will probably closely resemble an exposure technique, as the client must face a fear-producing situation to test an alternative way of thinking and its outcome.

Additional points that could be made:

a. The client is beginning to challenge the accuracy of the predictions that the fear generates, and the therapist suggests the client substitute more realistic self-talk. This is an important but difficult step for clients to make—there is resistance to change.

b. The therapist could have asked the client to provide alternative predictions rather than providing them for the client to consider. In later sessions the therapist will need to give this responsibility to the client.

c. Asking the client for other examples of faulty emotional reasoning from her own experience would help to drive home the unreliability of this pattern of thought.

Comments you would like to make:

_____

_____

_____

_____

Homework: The exercise "Negative Thoughts Trigger Negative Feelings" (*Adult Psychotherapy Homework Planner*, 2nd ed., by Jongsma) is an example of an intervention consistent with cognitive therapy that is designed to help educate the client about biased thinking and its impact on emotions. This assignment also provides opportunity for the client to examine her thinking in response to events in her life and begin to develop positive, reality-based replacement thoughts. Additional homework exercises consistent with cognitive restructuring are "Positive Self-Talk", "Journal and Replace Self-Defeating Thoughts," and "Journal of Distorted, Negative Thoughts" (see www.wiley.com/go/OCDwb).

Cognitive Therapy Review

1. What are the central elements of the cognitive therapy process?
2. What are common cognitive biases seen in OCD?

Cognitive Therapy Review Test Question

1 Kevin ritualistically prays for hours a day. He believes that if he doesn't, harm will come to his loved ones. Because of his need to pray, he has been unable to

hold a job. He spends most of his day at home. Which cognitive bias is prominent in Kevin's belief that he must keep praying?

A. Believing that thinking is the same as doing (thought-action fusion)
B. Inflating one's sense of personal responsibility
C. Overestimating the severity of the feared outcome
D. Underestimating one's capacity to manage a feared outcome

Exposure and Response Prevention

Exposure asks clients to engage repeatedly in what they fear, allowing the learned fear to extinguish over time. With OCD, it has been found that exposure works best when used with response (or ritual) prevention. Generally speaking, response prevention asks the client to refrain from engaging in his or her rituals once he/she has begun exposure to the triggers that have previously prompted the rituals. Exposures are typically guided by a hierarchy in which less-feared activities are conducted first. Imaginal exposure, live (or *in vivo*) exposure, or both may be used in treating OCD. Imaginal exposure typically involves imagining an obsessive thought or image or its feared consequences, allowing the emotion attached to the image to weaken. Exposure *in vivo* involves asking the client to actually engage in the activity he or she fears.

Key Points

SUMMARY OF CENTRAL ELEMENTS OF EXPOSURE AND RESPONSE PREVENTION

- Exposure asks clients to engage repeatedly in what they fear, allowing new learning to extinguish old (OCD-driven) learning over time.
- Response prevention asks the client to refrain from engaging in his/her rituals.
- Exposures are typically guided by a fear hierarchy.
- Imaginal exposure, live (or *in vivo*) exposure, or both may be used in treating OCD.
    - Imaginal exposure typically involves imagining an obsessive thought or image or its feared consequences.
    - Exposure *in vivo* involves asking the client to engage in the actual activity he or she fears.

Table 5.4 contains examples of an exposure/response prevention objective and interventions for OCD.

Table 5.4   Exposure/Response Prevention Objective and Interventions

Objective	Interventions
6. Undergo repeated imaginal or *in vivo* exposure to feared external and/or internal cues.	1. Direct and assist the client in construction of a hierarchy of feared internal and external fear cues. 2. Assess the nature of any external cues (e.g., persons, objects, and situations) and internal cues (thoughts, images, and impulses) that precipitate the client's obsessions and compulsions. 3. Select initial exposures (imaginal or *in vivo*) to the internal and/or external OCD cues that have a high likelihood of being a successful experience for the client; include response prevention and do cognitive restructuring within and after the exposure (see *Mastery of Obsessive-Compulsive Disorder* by Kozak & Foa; or *Treatment of Obsessive-Compulsive Disorder* by McGinn & Sanderson). 4. Assign the client a homework exercise in which he/she repeats the exposure to the internal and/or external OCD cues using response prevention and restructured cognitions between sessions and records responses (or assign "Reducing the Strength of Compulsive Behaviors" in *Adult Psychotherapy Homework Planner*, 2nd ed., by Jongsma); review during next session, reinforcing success and providing corrective feedback toward improvement (see *Mastery of Obsessive-Compulsive Disorder* by Kozak & Foa).

Demonstration Vignette
Exposure

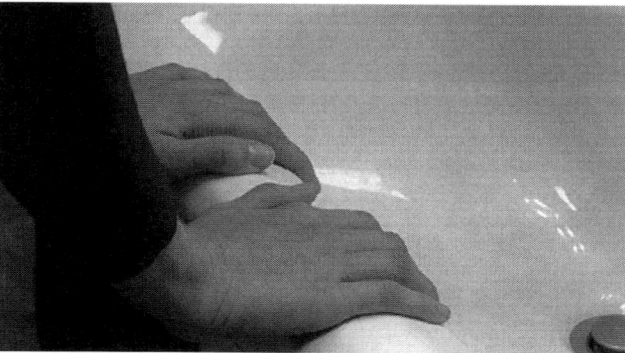

(continued)

Here we present the transcript of the dialogue depicted in the exposure therapy vignette.

Therapist: How are you feeling today, Jan?

Client: Nervous. Pretty nervous.

Therapist: About doing the exposure?

Client: Yeah.

Therapist: Well, that's perfectly normal. I'm glad you decided to do it. We're going to do this together and at your pace. It might be helpful to go over again why we're doing this. What's your sense of it?

Client: I think I need to prove to myself that my fears aren't true. I've felt better when I see that.

Therapist: Good. One of the ways we're going to do that is by testing the predictions we've generated, one set based on the fear, and the other based in reality, correcting for the biases associated with the fear.

Client: Yeah. When I look at them, I can kind of see that the fear looks exaggerated. It's just the nervousness, you know.

Therapist: I understand. Well, another reason for doing exposure is to allow that anxiety to run its course, to drain away. If we let it come on, ride it out without trying to run, it will weaken. As we do this repeatedly, we can expect the anxiety to diminish.

Client: I hope so.

Therapist: Good. Why don't we rehearse exactly what we're going to do before we try it?

Client: Okay.

Later in the session
[In the office restroom, standing in front of a sink]

Therapist: Okay Jan, we're going to work on exposure to the fears that you have from germs in the bathroom. Like we said, you're going to touch the surface of the sink and then just let your hands be—no wiping, rubbing, washing, just let them be. Just like we rehearsed, okay?

Client: Okay.

Therapist: While we're doing this, I'm going to ask you for your anxiety rating every once in a while so we can see what it's doing.

Client: Okay.

Therapist: And we're going to stay with it until the anxiety goes down noticeably. You and I will be talking about that throughout.

Client: All right.

Therapist: You ready?

Client: Yeah.

Therapist: Okay, also like we rehearsed, I'm going to show you what I'd like you to do, and then I'm going to ask you to do it, all right?

Client: All right.

Therapist: Okay, here we go. [The therapist places both hands on the countertop and then takes them off, describing what he/she is doing as he/she does it. He/she does not rub or wipe them. The client cringes some.]

Therapist: Okay, Jan, you ready?

Client: No, but I'm just going to do it.

Therapist: Good! What's your rating?

Client: 6 or 7.

Therapist: Okay, your turn.

[The client does the same thing, while the therapist encourages and praises the client for taking the challenge]

Therapist: Good job!

[Client sighs, looks somewhat uncomfortable, holding hands in front of them]

Therapist: Good job, Jan. What are you feeling?

Client: don't like it. I just feel like I'm contaminated.

Therapist: know. Hang in there. You're doing great! Where's your anxiety level now?

Client: Same, about a 6.

Therapist: Okay. How strong are your urges to clean your hands?

Client: Pretty strong—a 7 or 8.

Therapist: All right. You're doing just fine. Don't wash. Like we said, the anxiety and the urges are going to come, and your fear is going to want to talk to you. What's running through your head right now?

Client: I'm trying to stay strong, but then I just feel like I have germs crawling on me.

Therapist: Well, we knew you'd feel that way, that's not a surprise, and we know that we may or may not have some germs on us. Do you believe the germs are going to make you sick?

Client: Yes. I mean that's what I feel. I know it exaggerates, but that's what I feel.

Therapist: It does exaggerate, but it can make you feel like you do now. Does the feeling make it true?

Client: No, it doesn't. I'm trying to tell myself that.

Therapist: It's hard to believe that right now, isn't it?

Client: Yeah. It's not easy to see that it isn't true when I am in the middle of the fear. [Sighs deeply—calming a little]

Therapist: You're doing well. What's your rating?

Client: A 5 maybe. It's a little better.

Therapist: You seem less anxious. Where are you at now?

Client: Yeah, about a 3. I don't know. I think just talking about how it's just my fear talking to me, it helps me kind of stand apart from it.

Therapist: More like an observer, more objective?

Client: Yeah.

Therapist: Good. You're doing very well Jan.

Client: It does come down, doesn't it?

(*continued*)

Therapist:	Yeah. It may take longer or shorter depending on the task, but if you let it be and don't run from it by washing or something, it begins running out of steam.
Client:	But now we wait to see if I get sick.
Therapist:	Yeah, if *we* get sick.
Client:	Right.
Therapist:	And if we do, what are we going to do?
Client:	I know, just be sick.
Therapist:	What's your rating, Jan?
Client:	I'm feeling better. It's about a 2.
Therapist:	Very good. The unrealistic fear is fading.

Critique of the Exposure Demonstration Vignette

The following points were made in the critique:

a. The therapist makes good and frequent use of words of encouragement and reinforcement, such as, "You're doing very well."

b. The exposure is a behavioral technique, but there certainly is a cognitive restructuring component shown here, too. The client is testing predictions made from the fear as well as experiencing extinction of the fear through exposure.

c. The therapist gives a good explanation of the rationale of testing predictions generated by the underlying thoughts—an example of psychoeducation.

d. Rehearsal of the exposure is done in an office session before *in vivo* is implemented.

e. The therapist uses modeling first in the *in vivo* work and then couples the client's implementation with lots of encouragement and reinforcement of small steps of progress.

f. This represents a very early exposure experience, with more difficult sessions to follow.

Additional points that could be made:

a. The therapist made good use of humor to disarm the client and lower anxiety levels when he suggested he would be getting sick too if the client's dysfunctional prediction was accurate.

b. Repetition of this exposure a few times with decreasing levels of anxiety will lead to exposure to other items on the client's hierarchy of feared stimulus situations.

Comments you would like to make:

_____

_____

_____

_____

Homework: The homework exercise "Gradually Reducing Your Phobic Fear" (*Adult Psychotherapy Homework Planner* 2nd ed., by Jongsma) is an intervention that leads the client through the construction of an exposure hierarchy and exposure experience (see www.wiley.com/go/OCDwb).

Exposure Review

1. Define and describe exposure and response (or ritual) prevention.

Exposure Review Test Question

1 A client obsesses that he may harm someone while driving through residential areas. In the past, he would repeatedly circle areas to see if anyone had been hurt. In exposure and response prevention, this client would be asked to do which of the following?

   A. Discuss the actual likelihood of harming someone while driving
   B. Drive through a residential area without circling to check
   C. Imagine driving while pairing the image with a deep state of relaxation
   D. Not drive in residential areas

Chapter Reference

Jongsma, A. E. (2006). *Adult psychotherapy homework planner* (2nd ed.). Hoboken, NJ: Wiley.

6

What Are Considerations for Relapse Prevention?

Whether treated pharmacologically, psychologically, or both, obsessive-compulsive disorder can relapse. Let's take a look at some common considerations in relapse prevention interventions and how they can be incorporated into your treatment plan. With OCD, there is some empirical evidence supporting a more structured application of these interventions (e.g., Hiss, Foa, & Kozak, 1994).

1. Provide a rationale for relapse prevention that discusses the risk and introduces strategies for preventing it.
   ➤ One of the first steps in relapse prevention interventions is to provide a *rationale* for them. This typically involves a discussion of the risk for relapse and how using the relapse prevention approach we will outline can lower that risk.
2. Discuss with the client the distinction between a *lapse* and *relapse*, associating a lapse with a temporary setback and relapse with a return to a sustained pattern of depressive thinking, feeling, interpersonal withdrawal and/or avoidance.
   ➤ A lapse is presented as a rather common, temporary setback that may involve, for example, re-experiencing an obsessional thought, image, or impulse, or finding oneself engaging in an old compulsive behavior or mental act.
   ➤ Relapse, on the other hand, is described as a return to a sustained pattern of thinking, feeling, and acting that is characteristic of OCD.
   ➤ The rationale for this distinction is that lapses do not need to develop into a relapse if they can be caught and managed.
3. Identify and rehearse managing high-risk situations for a lapse.
   ➤ High-risk situations that might make the client vulnerable to a lapse are identified. This discussion may be informed by past difficult experiences or anticipated new ones. Some examples include:
      ➤ Having an interpersonal conflict after not having had one for some time
      ➤ Going to a new place where exposure hasn't been done, or being in the presence of old triggers for it

➤ Having a stressful day, week, or other period and starting to obsess or ritualize to ease the stress

➤ For the high-risk situations identified, the therapist leads the client in a rehearsal of using skills learned in therapy to manage them, including the skills of developing a tolerance for the lapse while working on how to begin problem-solving them.

4. Instruct the client to routinely use strategies learned in therapy, building them into his/her life as much as possible.

➤ In addition to using skills learned in therapy to manage high-risk situations, clients are also encouraged to use strategies learned in therapy during their day-to-day lives. Examples include everyday exposures, self-statements reflecting the new messages gained through cognitive restructuring, and problem-solving.

5. Develop a coping card on which coping strategies and other important information are kept.

➤ Sometimes clients benefit from having a coping card or some other reminder of important strategies and information regarding relapse prevention.

6. Schedule periodic maintenance or "booster" sessions to help the client maintain therapeutic gains and problem-solve challenges.

➤ Periodic "booster" sessions of therapy can help reinforce positive changes, problem-solve challenges, and facilitate continued improvement, so clients are invited to periodically revisit therapy for these purposes.

Common Considerations in Relapse Prevention

1. Explain the rationale of relapse prevention interventions
2. Distinguish between lapse and relapse
3. Identify and rehearse managing high-risk situations for a lapse
4. Encourage routine use of skills learned in therapy
5. Consider developing a coping card
6. Schedule periodic "booster" therapy sessions

Table 6.1 contains examples of how common considerations in relapse prevention could be incorporated into a psychotherapy treatment plan.

Table 6.1 Integrating Relapse Prevention Objective and Interventions into the Treatment Plan

Objective	Interventions
1. Learn and implement strategies to prevent relapse of obsessive-compulsive disorder.	1. Provide a rationale for relapse prevention that discusses the risk and introduces strategies for preventing it. 2. Discuss with the client the distinction between a lapse and relapse, associating a lapse with a temporary setback and relapse with a return to a sustained pattern of thinking, feeling, and behaving that is characteristic of OCD. 3. Identify and rehearse the management of future situations or circumstances in which lapses could occur. 4. Instruct the client to routinely use strategies learned in therapy (e.g., continued everyday exposure, cognitive restructuring, problem-solving), building them into his/her life as much as possible. 5. Develop a coping card on which coping strategies and other important information can be kept (e.g., guidelines for exposure, positive coping statements, other reminders that were helpful to the client during therapy). 6. Schedule periodic maintenance or "booster" sessions to help the client maintain therapeutic gains and problem-solve challenges.

Demonstration Vignette

Relapse Prevention

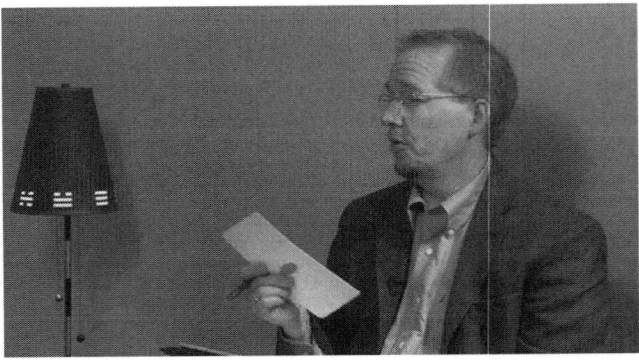

Here we present the transcript of the dialogue depicted in the OCD relapse prevention vignette.

Therapist: Jan, last time we talked about how some people who have overcome OCD are still vulnerable to having a lapse, where they find themselves obsessing about something or ritualizing after not having not done so for awhile.

Client: Right, I remember.

Therapist: Good. You may also recall that we made a distinction between a lapse or setback and a "relapse," which involves reverting back to having fear and avoidance guide your daily actions more completely—like when you first came in for treatment.

Client: I can't imagine going back to that, but I think it's good to know what I should be doing to prevent it.

Therapist: Great, that's what I'd like to spend some time with today. So let's start with stress. It's not unusual for lapses to occur while we're under stress. The stress could be general everyday things; it could be a particularly demanding situation, like increased demands at work, or it might be a situation that used to be associated with the OCD—where you may feel a pull to go back to the old habits.

Client: Okay. I can see that.

Therapist: So, why don't we begin by looking into the near future, identifying any foreseeable challenges—situations that might challenge you to forget what you learned in therapy?

Client: Okay. Well one thing that's been on my mind is the upcoming holidays. We'll stay over with my husband's family for a few days. Being away from home, all the different people, using their restrooms, of course. I haven't done that in awhile and I've been thinking about how I'm going to do there.

Therapist: That's a great example. You haven't done that in awhile. So, let's imagine going to your relatives' house, like a rehearsal of it, and walk through what you want to try to do to meet the challenges you anticipate.

Therapist: Let's talk a little about a different type of challenge and what you want to do should it come up. Let's imagine you've discovered that you've actually had a setback, and let's talk about what you want to try to do should that occur.

Client: You mean like if I started washing again?

Therapist: Yeah, or found yourself starting to be consumed with the thought of contamination. Maybe work has been busy and you're feeling stressed.

Client: Okay. That definitely happens.

Therapist: All right. And imagine under the stress of that, you find yourself starting to wash excessively, kind of mindlessly, and you find yourself thinking about it again. . . . Maybe you've done it a few times and then realize you've had this little setback. Let's talk about what you want to try to do to get back on track.

Client: All right. Well, the first thing that comes to my mind is to get a handle on my thinking . . .

Therapist: All right, Jan, so let's review what you want to try to do should you have a setback. I'm going to write them down on this coping card that you can take with you as a reminder if you ever need it.

Client: Okay, good. Well, first I'd talk to myself, put things in perspective.

Therapist: Say things like what?

Client: Things like: "This is what we said could occur. It's not a catastrophe. It is not a relapse." And just remind myself that I've managed this before.

(continued)

Therapist: Excellent! And we want to not let it spread to other situations, right.

Client: Right, "Restrict the setback."

Therapist: Exactly. And then what? How do you want to proceed from there?

Client: Well, I like the idea of rewinding the tape and thinking about how I would do it again.

Therapist: Okay. Kind of a "do-over" in your mind.

Client: Yeah. And then plan it out—how I want to do it next time.

Therapist: Good, lay out how you want to do it. And then?

Client: And then, go do it.

Therapist: Excellent, Jan. And do you want to add any memory aids, like on sinks or mirrors for this?

Client: Yeah, I still have the little blue dots all over the place. They'd help remind me of my plan.

Therapist: Great! How about a few self-statements on the card that help you stay strong?

Client: I think we can just put that: "Be strong. Be positive. Be realistic."

Therapist: What do those words mean for you?

Client: It's kind of what I have said to myself to help me get through the exposures we've done. I used to say it before all this, whenever I needed a boost.

Therapist: So, it's coming back to you? It's believable again?

Client: Yeah. It makes me feel good about myself.

Critique of the Relapse Prevention Demonstration Vignette

The following points were made in the critique:

  a. The therapist helped the client identify high-risk situations for relapse and points out how stress increases vulnerability to lapse.

  b. The therapist reviewed several coping skills that may help the client avoid relapse (e.g., self talk, "rewind the tape," relaxation, a coping card of positive messages, such as, "be strong, be positive, be realistic").

  c. Memory aids can help the client remember positive self-talk, and "blue dots" placed in the environment can trigger positive thoughts.

Additional points that could be made:

  a. The therapist reviewed the positive self-talk messages the client has used before and those that she can use in future high-risk situations.

  b. The therapist makes good use of rehearsal to strengthen the client's confidence in facing feared situations.

  c. The therapist uses a psychoeducation review to drive home the difference between a lapse and relapse. This is another way to strengthen the client for the weeks ahead.

Comments you would like to make:

_____

_____

_____

_____

Homework: The assignment "Applying Problem-Solving to Interpersonal Conflict" is an exercise that leads the client through seven steps of problem solving. These steps can be applied to various problems the client encounters, and this skill is important in helping to prevent relapse. The exercise "Journal and Replace Self-Defeating Thoughts" reinforces the client's knowledge regarding cognitive biases that can lead to relapse (see www.wiley.com/go/OCDwb).

Chapter Review

1. What are the common considerations in relapse prevention?

Chapter Review Test Question

1. James is nearing the end of his treatment for OCD. For several weeks he has been doing exposure and response prevention successfully. His therapist gives him a homework assignment that asks him to list future situations that might challenge him to revert back to his old OCD habits. They plan to review the list and develop a plan for managing the challenges effectively. Which consideration in relapse prevention is depicted in this example?

    A. Developing a coping card
    B. Distinguishing between lapse and relapse
    C. Encouraging routine use of skills learned in therapy
    D. Identifying high-risk situations for a lapse

Chapter References

Eisen, J. L., Goodman, W. K., Keller, M. B., Warshaw, M. G., DeMarco, L. M., Luce, D. D., & Rasmussen, S. A. (1999). Patterns of remission and relapse in obsessive-compulsive disorder: A 2-year prospective study. *Journal of Clinical Psychiatry, 60,* 346–351.

Hiss, H., Foa, E. B., & Kozak, M. J. (1994). A relapse prevention program for treatment of obsessive-compulsive disorder. *Journal of Consulting and Clinical Psychology, 62,* 801–808.

Closing Remarks and Resources

As we note on the DVD, it is important to be aware that the research support for any particular EST supports the identified treatment as it was delivered in the empirical studies. The use of only selected objectives or interventions from ESTs may not be empirically supported.

If you want to incorporate an EST into your treatment plan, it should reflect the major objectives and interventions of the approach. Note that in addition to their primary objectives and interventions, many ESTs have options within them that may or may not be used depending on the client's need (e.g., skills training). Most treatment manuals, books, and other training programs identify the primary objectives and interventions used in the EST.

An existing resource for integrating research-supported treatments into treatment planning is the Practice*Planners*® Series[1] of treatment planners. The series contains several books that have integrated goals, objectives, and interventions consistent with those of identified ESTs into treatment plans for several applicable problems and disorders:

➤ *The Severe and Persistent Mental Illness Treatment Planner* (Berghuis, Jongsma, & Bruce)
➤ *The Family Therapy Treatment Planner* (Dattilio, Jongsma, & Davis)
➤ *The Complete Adult Psychotherapy Treatment Planner* (Jongsma, Peterson, & Bruce)
➤ *The Adolescent Psychotherapy Treatment Planner* (Jongsma, Peterson, McInnis, & Bruce)
➤ *The Child Psychotherapy Treatment Planner* (Jongsma, Peterson, McInnis, & Bruce)

---

[1]These books are updated frequently; please check with the publisher for the latest editions and for further information about the Practice *Planners*® series.

➤ *The Veterans and Active Duty Military Psychotherapy Treatment Planner* (Moore & Jongsma)

➤ *The Addiction Treatment Planner* (Perkinson, Jongsma, & Bruce)

➤ *The Couples Psychotherapy Treatment Planner* (O'Leary, Heyman, & Jongsma)

➤ *The Older Adult Psychotherapy Treatment Planner* (Frazer, Hinrichsen, & Jongsma).

Finally, it is important to remember that the purpose of this series is to demonstrate the process of evidence-based psychotherapy treatment planning for common mental health problems. It is designed to be informational in nature, and does not intend to be a substitute for clinical training in the interventions discussed and demonstrated. In accordance with ethical guidelines, therapists should have competency in the services they deliver.

A

A Sample Evidence-Based Treatment Plan for Obsessive-Compulsive Disorder

Primary Problem: Obsessive-Compulsive Disorder (OCD)

Behavioral Definitions:

1. Intrusive, recurrent, and unwanted thoughts, images, or impulses that distress and/or interfere with the client's daily routine, job performance, or social relationships
2. Failed attempts to ignore or control these thoughts or impulses or to neutralize them with other thoughts and actions
3. Recognition that obsessive thoughts are a product of his/her own mind
4. Repetitive and/or excessive mental or behavioral actions done to neutralize or prevent discomfort or some dreaded outcome
5. Recognition of repetitive thoughts and/or behaviors as being excessive and unreasonable—not realistic worries about life's problems

Diagnosis: Obsessive-Compulsive Disorder (300.3)

Long-Term Goals:

1. Reduce the frequency, intensity, and duration of obsessions and compulsions
2. Function daily at a consistent level with minimal interference from obsessions and compulsions

Objectives	Interventions
1. Describe the nature and history of OCD symptoms.	1. Focus on developing a level of trust with the client; provide support and empathy to encourage the client to feel safe in expressing his/her OCD symptoms. 2. Assess the client's frequency, intensity, duration, and history of obsessions and compulsions (e.g., *The Anxiety Disorders Interview Schedule for the DSM-IV* by DiNardo, Brown, & Barlow).
2. Complete psychological testing or objective questionnaires for assessing OCD.	1. Administer an objective test of OCD symptoms to further assess its depth and breadth (e.g., *The Yale-Brown Obsessive Compulsive Scale* by Goodman et. al.)

(continued)

Objectives	Interventions
3. Obtain a complete medical evaluation to rule out medical- and substance-related causes for anxiety symptoms.	1. Refer the client to a general physician for a complete medical examination to rule out medical- or substance-related etiology for the anxiety. 2. Assist the client in following up on the recommendations from a physical evaluation, including medications, lab work, or specialty assessments.
4. Cooperate with a medication evaluation.	1. Assess the client's need for medication (e.g., selective serotonin reuptake inhibitors). 2. Monitor and evaluate the client's psychotropic medication prescription compliance and the effectiveness of the medication on his/her level of functioning.
5. Keep a daily journal of obsessions, compulsions, and triggers; record thoughts, feelings, and actions taken.	1. Ask the client to keep a daily journal in which he/she documents obsessions, compulsions, and triggers and records thoughts, feelings, and actions taken; routinely process the journal toward helping the client understand his/her contributions to generating his/her anger.
6. Verbalize an accurate understanding of PTSD and how it develops.	1. Convey a cognitive behavioral model for the development and maintenance of OCD, highlighting the role of fears and avoidance in its maintenance (see *Mastery of Obsessive-Compulsive Disorder* by Kozak & Foa).
7. Verbalize an understanding of the treatment rationale for PTSD.	1. Discuss how treatment serves as an arena to desensitize learned fear, reality-test obsessional fears and underlying beliefs, and build confidence in managing fears without compulsions (see *Mastery of Obsessive-Compulsive Disorder* by Kozak & Foa). 2. Assign the client to read psychoeducational chapters of books or treatment manuals on the rationale for exposure and ritual prevention therapy and/or cognitive restructuring for OCD (e.g., *Mastery of Obsessive-Compulsive Disorder* by Foa & Kozak or *Stop Obsessing* by Foa & Wilson).
8. Identify and replace biased, fearful self-talk and beliefs.	1. Explore the client's biased schema and self-talk that mediate his/her obsessional fears and compulsions; assist him/her in generating thoughts that correct for the biases; use behavioral experiments to test fearful versus alternative predictions (see *Obsessive-Compulsive Disorder* by Salkovskis & Kirk). 2. Assign the client a homework exercise in which he/she identifies fearful self-talk, identifies biases in the self-talk, generates alternatives, and tests through behavioral experiments; review and reinforce success, providing corrective feedback toward improvement.

Objectives	Interventions
9. Undergo repeated imaginal or *in vivo* exposure to feared internal and/or external cues.	1. Assess the nature of any internal cues (thoughts, images, and impulses) and external cues (e.g., persons, objects, and situations) that precipitate the client's obsessions and compulsions. 2. Direct and assist the client in construction of fear hierarchies related to feared internal and external fear cues. 3. Conduct initial exposures (imaginal or *in vivo*) to the internal and/or external OCD cues that have a high likelihood of being a successful experience for the client; include response prevention and do cognitive restructuring within and after the exposure (see *Mastery of Obsessive-Compulsive Disorder* by Kozak and Foa or *Treatment of Obsessive-Compulsive Disorder* by McGinn & Sanderson). 4. Assign the client a homework exercise in which he/she repeats the exposure to the internal and/or external OCD cues using response prevention and restructured cognitions between sessions and records responses (or assign "Reducing the Strength of Compulsive Behaviors" in *Adult Psychotherapy Homework Planner*, 2nd ed., by Jongsma); review during next session, reinforcing success and providing corrective feedback toward improvement (see *Mastery of Obsessive-Compulsive Disorder* by Foa & Kozak).
10. Learn and implement strategies to prevent relapse of OCD.	1. Provide a rationale for relapse prevention that discusses the risk and introduces strategies for preventing it. 2. Discuss with the client the distinction between a lapse and relapse, associating a lapse with a temporary setback and relapse with a return to a sustained pattern of thinking, feeling, and behaving that is characteristic of OCD. 3. Identify and rehearse the management of future situations or circumstances in which lapses could occur. 4. Instruct the client to routinely use strategies learned in therapy (e.g., continued everyday exposure, cognitive restructuring, problem-solving), building them into his/her life as much as possible. 5. Develop a coping card on which coping strategies and other important information can be kept (e.g., steps in problem-solving, positive coping statements, reminders that were helpful to the client during therapy). 6. Schedule periodic maintenance or "booster" sessions to help the client maintain therapeutic gains and problem-solve challenges.

B

Chapter Review Test Questions and Answers Explained

Chapter 1: What is Obsessive–Compulsive Disorder?

1. Which of the following best reflects the definition of obsessions, according to diagnostic criteria such as those of the DSM?

    A. Recurrent and persistent images
    B. Recurrent and persistent impulses
    C. Recurrent and persistent thoughts
    D. Recurrent and persistent thoughts, images, or impulses

    A. *Incorrect*: Obsessions are not restricted to images only.
    B. *Incorrect*: Obsessions are not restricted to impulses only.
    C. *Incorrect*: Obsessions are not restricted to thoughts only.
    D. *Correct*: Obsessions can be thoughts, images, or impulses.

2. Which of the following describes common compulsions?

    A. Aggressive impulses and images
    B. Checking and washing
    C. Contamination fears and washing
    D. Harming fears and reassurance seeking

    A. *Incorrect*: Impulses and images are obsessions, not compulsions.
    B. *Correct*: Repeated checking and washing are examples of common compulsions.
    C. *Incorrect*: Although washing is a common compulsion, fears surrounding contamination are a common obsessional theme.
    D. *Incorrect*: Although reassurance seeking is a common compulsion, fear of harming someone in some way is a common obsessional theme.

Chapter 2: What Are the Six Steps in Building a Treatment Plan?

1. Persons with obsessive-compulsive disorder may engage in compulsive acts that, although meeting the criteria for a compulsion, are particular to that individual's beliefs regarding how they work. Examples include performing acts in threes, hoarding only certain types of objects, and washing a certain way for a certain length of time. In which step of treatment planning would you record these features of your particular client?

   A. Creating short-term objectives
   B. Describing the problem's manifestations
   C. Identifying the primary problem
   D. Selecting treatment interventions
      A. *Incorrect*: Particular compulsions are a feature or symptom manifestation, not an objective for the client to achieve.
      B. *Correct*: Features, also referred to as behavioral definitions, expressions, or manifestations, of a problem for the particular client are described in Step 2 of treatment planning: Describing the problem's manifestations.
      C. *Incorrect*: Particular compulsions are a feature or symptom manifestation of the primary problem of OCD.
      D. *Incorrect*: Particular compulsions are a feature or symptom manifestation, not a therapist's action designed to help the client achieve his or her objective(s).

2. The statement "Discuss with the client how treatment serves as an arena to desensitize learned fear, reality-test obsessional fears and underlying beliefs, and build confidence in managing fears without compulsions," is an example of which of the following features of a treatment plan?

   A. A primary problem
   B. A short-term objective
   C. A symptom manifestation
   D. A treatment intervention
      A. *Incorrect*: The primary problem (Step 1 in Treatment Planning) is the summary description, usually in diagnostic terms, of the client's primary problem.
      B. *Incorrect*: Short-term objectives (Step 5 in Treatment Planning) describe the desired actions of the client in the treatment plan.
      C. *Incorrect*: Symptom manifestations (Step 2 in Treatment Planning) describe the client's particular expression (i.e., manifestations or symptoms) of a problem.

D. *Correct*: A treatment intervention (Step 6 in Treatment Planning) describes the therapist's actions designed to help the client achieve therapeutic objectives.

Chapter 3: What Is the Brief History of the Empirically Supported Treatments Movement?

1   Which statement best describes the process used to identify ESTs?

A. Consumers of mental health services nominated therapies.
B. Experts came to a consensus based on their experiences with the treatments.
C. Researchers submitted their works.
D. Task groups reviewed the literature using clearly defined selection criteria for ESTs.

  A. *Incorrect*: Mental health professionals selected ESTs.
  B. *Incorrect*: Expert consensus was not the method used to identify ESTs.
  C. *Incorrect*: Empirical works in the existing literature were reviewed to identify ESTs.
  D. *Correct*: Review groups consisting of mental health professionals selected ESTs based on predetermined criteria such as *well-established* and *probably efficacious*.

2. Based on the differences in their criteria, in which of the following ways are well-established treatments different than those classified as probably efficacious?

A. Only the probably efficacious criteria allowed the use of a single case design experiments.
B. Only the well-established criteria allowed studies comparing the treatment to a psychological placebo.
C. Only the well-established criteria required demonstration by at least two different, independent investigators or investigating teams.
D. Only the well-established criteria allowed studies comparing the treatment to a pill placebo.

  A. *Incorrect*: Both sets of criteria allowed use of single subject designs. Well-established treatments required a larger series than did probably efficacious treatments (see II under Well-Established and III under Probably Efficacious).
  B. *Incorrect*: Studies using comparison to psychological placebos were acceptable in both sets of criteria (see IA under Well-Established and II under Probably Efficacious).

    C. *Correct*: One of the primary differences between treatments classified as well-established and those classified as probably efficacious is that well-established therapies have had their efficacy demonstrated by at least two different, independent investigators (see V under Well-Established).

    D. *Incorrect*: Studies using comparison to pill placebos were acceptable in both sets of criteria (see IA under Well-Established and II under Probably Efficacious).

Chapter 4: What are the Identified Empirically Supported Treatments for Obsessive–Compulsive Disorder?

1. Cognitive behavioral therapy (CBT) that includes which of the following is a well-established treatment for OCD and the recommended first-line psychotherapeutic treatment option in evidence-based practice guidelines?

    A. Exposure and response prevention (ERP)

    B. Psychoeducation (PE)

    C. Relaxation training (RT)

    D. Systematic desensitization (SD)

        A. *Correct*: Several reviewers and evidence-based practice guidelines cite CBT with ERP as a well-established treatment for OCD.

        B. *Incorrect*: Although initial and ongoing PE is a common feature of CBT with ERP, it is not a well-established treatment for OCD in and of itself.

        C. *Incorrect*: Although RT may be taught within CBT with ERP, it is not a well-established treatment for OCD in and of itself.

        D. *Incorrect*: Although SD was an early treatment for anxiety-based problems that is still used today in some applications, it is not a well-established treatment for OCD.

2. Asking a client with OCD to stop or limit compulsive rituals associated with an exposure is known as which of the following?

    A. Behavioral experiment

    B. Cognitive restructuring

    C. Limit setting

    D. Response prevention

        A. *Incorrect*: A behavioral experiment is a cognitive therapy technique that involves treating beliefs as hypotheses and testing their validity in one's experience.

B. *Incorrect*: Cognitive restructuring is a broad term from cognitive therapy that describes the process of identifying, challenging, and changing maladaptive thoughts, beliefs, or underlying assumptions.

C. *Incorrect*: Although used generally in several applications, limit setting is a technique commonly seen in therapies involving children (e.g., play therapy) where behavioral boundaries or limits are establishing for specific activities.

D. *Correct*: Response prevention refers to limiting or eliminating compulsions in conjunction with a particular exposure. It has been shown to be an important component of exposure-based treatment for OCD.

Chapter 5: How Do You Integrate Empirically Supported Treatments into Treatment Planning?

Assessment/Psychoeducation

1. At what point in therapy is psychoeducation typically conducted?
   A. At the end of therapy
   B. During the assessment phase
   C. During the initial treatment session
   D. Throughout therapy
      A. *Incorrect*: Psychoeducation is done throughout therapy.
      B. *Incorrect*: Psychoeducation is done throughout therapy.
      C. *Incorrect*: Psychoeducation is done throughout therapy.
      D. *Correct*: Well, you know the answer.

Cognitive Therapy

1. Kevin ritualistically prays for hours a day. He believes that if he doesn't, harm will come to his loved ones. Because of his need to pray, he has been unable to hold a job. He spends most of his day at home. Which cognitive bias is prominent in Kevin's belief that he must keep praying?
   A. Believing that thinking is the same as doing (thought-action fusion)
   B. Inflating one's sense of personal responsibility
   C. Overestimating the severity of the feared outcome
   D. Underestimating one's capacity to manage a feared outcome
      A. *Incorrect*: This bias is more common in harming obsessions, in which the person believes that thinking the harming thought is like doing it. Kevin ritualizes to prevent an outcome.

      B. *Correct*: Kevin believes that he/his actions are personally responsible for preventing the bad outcome, which in fact would be influenced by several factors other than his actions.

      C. *Incorrect*: Although this bias is likely to be operating in Kevin's fear that the death of a loved one would be catastrophically severe, it is not directly responsible for maintaining his rituals.

      D. *Incorrect*: As with C, although this bias is likely to be operating in Kevin's fear that the death of a loved would be too difficult to manage, it is not directly responsible for maintaining his rituals.

Exposure

1. A client obsesses that he may harm someone while driving through residential areas. In the past, he would repeatedly circle areas to see if anyone had been hurt. In exposure and response prevention, this client would be asked to do which of the following?

  A. Discuss the actual likelihood of harming someone while driving

  B. Drive through a residential area without circling to check

  C. Imagine driving while pairing the image with a deep state of relaxation

  D. Not drive in residential areas

      A. *Incorrect*: This intervention is more consistent with cognitive therapy, but may be used in more integrative CBT.

      B. *Correct*: In exposure and response prevention, clients are asked to do the activity that they (unrealistically) believe will produce the feared outcome, while not engaging in the ritual it provokes.

      C. *Incorrect*: This is more consistent with systematic desensitization, than with exposure and response prevention.

      D. *Incorrect*: This is the antithesis of what an exposure therapist would do, as it is a form of avoidance that would maintain the fear.

Chapter 6: What Are Considerations for Relapse Prevention?

1. James is nearing the end of his treatment for OCD. For several weeks he has been doing exposure and response prevention successfully. His therapist gives him a homework assignment that asks him to list future situations that might challenge him to revert back to his old OCD habits. They plan to review the list and develop a plan for managing the challenges effectively. Which consideration in relapse prevention is depicted in this example?

A. Developing a coping card
B. Distinguishing between lapse and relapse
C. Encouraging routine use of skills learned in therapy
D. Identifying high-risk situations for a lapse

    A. *Incorrect*: This is a technique used by some clients to help them remember key therapeutic points and strategies outside of therapy.

    B. *Incorrect*: This is a psychoeducational intervention designed in part to help prevent misinterpretation of potentially manageable "setbacks" as an unmanageable relapse.

    C. *Incorrect*: This intervention is designed to transport skill use into everyday applications, not just ones that represent a higher risk for relapse.

    D. *Correct*: The vignette describes identifying high-risk situations. James and his therapist will then review and develop a plan for managing them.

STUDY PACKAGE
CONTINUING EDUCATION
CREDIT INFORMATION

Evidence-Based Treatment Planning for Obsessive-Compulsive Disorder

Our goal is to provide you with current, accurate and practical information from the most experienced and knowledgeable speakers and authors.

Listed below are the continuing education credit(s) currently available for this self-study package. *Please note: Your state licensing board dictates whether self study is an acceptable form of continuing education. Please refer to your state rules and regulations.*

COUNSELORS: PESI is recognized by the National Board for Certified Counselors to offer continuing education for National Certified Counselors. Provider #: 5896. We adhere to NBCC Continuing Education Guidelines This self-study package qualifies for **1.0** contact hours.

SOCIAL WORKERS: PESI, 1030, is approved as a provider for continuing education by the Association of Social Work Boards, 400 South Ridge Parkway, Suite B, Culpeper, VA 22701. www.aswb.org. Social workers should contact their regulatory board to determine course approval. Course Level: All Levels. Social Workers will receive **1.0** (Clinical) continuing education clock hours for completing this self-study package.

PSYCHOLOGISTS: PESI is approved by the American Psychological Association to sponsor continuing education for psychologists. PESI maintains responsibility for these materials and their content. PESI is offering these self- study materials for **1.0** hours of continuing education credit.

ADDICTION COUNSELORS: PESI is a Provider approved by NAADAC Approved Education Provider Program. Provider #: 366. This self-study package qualifies for **1.0** contact hours

Procedures:

       1. Review the material and read the book.

       2. If seeking credit, complete the posttest/evaluation form:

            -Complete posttest/evaluation in entirety; including your email address to receive your certificate much faster versus by mail.

            -Upon completion, mail to the address listed on the form along with the CE fee stated on the test. Tests will not be processed without the CE fee included.

            -Completed posttests must be received 6 months from the date printed on the packing slip.

Your completed posttest/evaluation will be graded. If you receive a passing score (70% and above), you will be emailed/faxed/mailed a certificate of successful completion with earned continuing education credits. (Please write your email address on the posttest/evaluation form for fastest response) If you do not pass the posttest, you will be sent a letter indicating areas of deficiency, and another posttest to complete. The posttest must be resubmitted and receive a passing grade before credit can be awarded. We will allow you to re-take as many times as necessary to receive a certificate.

If you have any questions, please feel free to contact our customer service department at 1.800.844.8260.

PESI LLC
PO BOX 1000
Eau Claire, WI 54702-1000

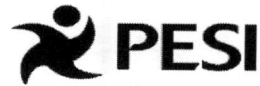 **PESI**

Evidence-Based Treatment Planning for Obsessive-Compulsive Disorder

PO BOX 1000
Eau Claire, WI 54702
800-844-8260

Any persons interested in receiving credit may photocopy this form, complete and return with a payment of $15.00 per person CE fee. A certificate of successful completion will be sent to you. To receive your certificate sooner than two weeks, rush processing is available for a fee of $10. Please attach check or include credit card information below.

Mail to: PESI, PO Box 1000, Eau Claire, WI 54702 or fax to PESI (800) 554-9775 (both sides)

CE Fee: $15: (Rush processing fee: $10)   **Total to be charged** _____

Credit Card #: _____ **Exp Date:** _____ **V-Code*:** _____
(*MC/VISA/Discover: last 3-digit # on signature panel on back of card.) (*American Express: 4-digit # above account # on face of card.)

	LAST	FIRST	M.I.

Name (please print): _____ _____ _____

Address: _____ Daytime Phone: _____

City: _____ State: _____ Zip Code: _____

Signature: _____ Email: _____

Date Completed: _____ Actual time (# of hours) taken to complete this offering: _____ hours

Program Objectives After completing this publication, I have been able to achieve these objectives:

1. Explain the process and criteria for diagnosing obsessive-compulsive disorder.   1. Yes   No

2. List the six steps in building a psychotherapy treatment plan.   2. Yes   No

3. Examine how empirically supported treatments for obsessive-compulsive disorder have been identified.   3. Yes   No

4. Examine the objectives and treatment interventions consistent with those of identified empirically supported treatments for obsessive-compulsive disorder.   4. Yes   No

5. Describe how to construct a psychotherapy treatment plan and inform it with objectives and treatment interventions identified empirically supported treatments for obsessive-compulsive disorder.   5. Yes   No

6. Identify common considerations in the prevention of relapse of obsessive-compulsive disorder.   6. Yes   No

PESI LLC
PO BOX 1000
Eau Claire, WI 54702-1000

ZNT043365

CE Release Date: 2/11/2011

Participant Profile:

1. Job Title: _____   Employment setting: _____

1. According to psychiatric classification system criteria for the diagnosis of obsessive-compulsive disorder, which of the following are recurrent and persistent thoughts, images, or impulses that are intrusive, inappropriate, cause marked anxiety or distress, and are recognized by the sufferer as a product of his or her own mind?
A. Compulsions
B. Delusions
C. Hallucinations
D. Obsessions

2. Obsessive-compulsive disorder is not diagnosed if an apparent obsession or compulsion is a primary feature of another mental disorder and restricted to it. Examples include the preoccupation with food within an eating disorder, or the concern with appearance within body dysmorphic disorder.
A. True
B. False

3. A psychotherapy treatment plan contains statements such as, "Experiences intrusive, recurrent and unwanted thoughts that interfere with the client's daily routine," "failed attempts to ignore or control these thoughts." These statements constitute which of the following elements of a psychotherapy treatment plan?
A. Behavioral definitions
B. Primary problems
C. Short-term objective
D. Therapeutic interventions

4. As discussed in this program, reviewers of the psychotherapy treatment outcome literature have identified which of the following treatments as having demonstrated efficacy in the treatment of obsessive-compulsive disorder?
A. Both cognitive therapy and exposure and response prevention
B. Cognitive therapy only
C. Exposure therapy only
D. Exposure and response prevention only

5. Response prevention is the act of repeatedly engaging in a fear activity until the anxiety associated with it diminishes.
A. True
B. False

6. In a research-supported therapy for obsessive compulsive disorder, a therapist asks her client to refrain from washing his hands for a specified period of time after the client has touched something he believes has contaminated them. The therapeutic instruction to refrain from washing is called what?
A. Cognitive therapy
B. Exposure and response prevention
C. Psychoeducation
D. Relapse prevention

7. Jim struggles with obsessive-compulsive disorder (OCD). He has experienced intrusive images of harming someone. He believes this means that he is actually likely to act on these images and therefore concludes that he must be a very bad person. His therapist discusses this interpretation with him exploring alternative interpretations and conclusions. This type of intervention is most characteristic of which research-supported treatment for OCD?
A. Cognitive therapy
B. Exposure and response prevention
C. Psychoeducation
D. Relapse prevention

8. Cognitive therapy and exposure and response prevention are often combined in a treatment approach generally referred to as cognitive behavioral therapy with exposure and response prevention (CBT with ERP).
A. True
B. False

9. According to this program, an intervention commonly used in relapse prevention is to identify and rehearse coping with high-risk times for relapse.
A. True
B. False

10. Which of the following best describes the approach to creating an evidence-based treatment plan for obsessive-compulsive disorder that is recommended in this program?
A. The therapist conducts cognitive therapy.
B. The therapist conducts exposure therapy.
C. The therapist incorporates into therapy the objectives and interventions consistent with research-supported treatments for obsessive-compulsive disorder.
D. The therapist uses an objective measure of obsessive-compulsive disorder to track treatment progress.

PESI LLC
PO BOX 1000
Eau Claire, WI 54702-1000